INTERNATIONAL CUISINE

Japan

Reiko Hara

Hod

www.h

Orders: please contact Bookpoint Ltd, 130 Milton Park, Abingdon, Oxon OX14 4SB. Telephone: (44) 01235 827720. Fax: (44) 01235 400454. Lines are open from 9.00 - 6.00, Monday to Saturday, with a 24 hour message answering service. You can also order through our website www.hoddereducation.co.uk.

If you have any comments to make about this, or any of our other titles, please send them to educationenquiries@hodder.co.uk

British Library Cataloguing in Publication Data
A catalogue record for this title is available from the British Library

ISBN-10: 0 340 905 778
ISBN-13: 978 0 340 905 777

First Edition Published 2006
This Edition Published 2006
Impression number 10 9 8 7 6 5 4 3 2 1
Year   2011 2010 2009 2008 2007 2006

Hodder Headline's policy is to use papers that are natural, renewable and recyclable products and made from wood grown in sustainable forests. The logging and manufacturing processes are expected to conform to the environmental regulations of the country of origin.

Cover photo by Sam Bailey

Illustrations by Richard Morris

Illustrations on p.13 from THE OKINAWA DIET PLAN by Bradley J. Willcox, M.D, D. Craig Willcox, PhD, and Makoto Suzuki, M.D, with Leah Feldon, copyright © 2004 by Bradley J. Willcox and D. Craig Willcox. Used by permission of Clarkson Potter/Publishers, a division of Random House, Inc.

Typeset by Pantek Arts Ltd, Maidstone Kent

Printed in Great Britain for Hodder Arnold, an imprint of Hodder Education, a member of the Hodder Headline Group, 338 Euston Road, London NW1 3BH

Contents

Foreword																		v
Acknowledgements														vi
Introduction															vii

## Section 1 Culture and Cuisine												1
  1 Geography															3
  2 Historical background												5
  3 The health benefits of Japanese food					11
  4 Menu planning													18

## Section 2 Tools and Ingredients											19
  5 Basic kitchen tools												21
  6 Techniques														25
  7 Initial preparation											38
  8 Ingredients														46

## Section 3 Recipes															69
  9 Getting started: beginners' recipes						71
10 Sushi																		91
11 Tofu																		105
12 Vegetables																	112
13 Eggs																		123
14 Fish																		128
15 Poultry																		142
16 Meat																		154
17 Rice																		167
18 Noodles																		175
19 Soups																		180
20 Pickles																		184
21 Desserts																	186

Useful addresses															189
Index																			193

Foreword

It gives me an immense pleasure to see Reiko's first book in print. This book encapsulates her life-long passion for cooking, encompassing European as well as Asian cooking, and her exceptional quality as a teacher.

Japanese cuisine has much to offer to Western chefs in its style, presentation and tastes. Its recent popularity surge, therefore, is not surprising, especially when it has an additional appeal of health benefits. In fact, in that sense, the cuisine with a more than 600-year history is uncannily modern.

At Thames Valley University, Reiko pioneered our first Japanese cookery courses aimed at professional as well as student chefs of diverse cultural backgrounds and experiences. In the classroom, she has repeatedly demonstrated her ability to communicate uniquely Japanese culinary concepts, often completely alien to Western chefs, with such clarity and ease. She has a focused and practical approach to cooking and a love of food which is infectious.

This book is a reflection of her accomplishments as a dedicated teacher of unique qualities and flair, which give it a unique place on the market. This book explains the basic principles of this relatively unexplored cuisine in a way that makes sense to Westerners, while providing its cultural and historical backgrounds, as well as its health benefits.

I hope this is only the first of many books Reiko will publish in what I hope will be her long and successful career as an educator and a chef with a truly global perspective.

Professor David Foskett MBE

Acknowledgements

The author wishes to thank the following people. Saburo and Motoko Hara, my parents, for encouraging me to write this book and, more importantly, for making me aware that eating well at home is fundamental to life. Professor David Foskett MBE for his support for the Asian Culinary Arts programme at Thames Valley University. Nobuko Hara for her brilliant work as editorial adviser. The Operations Department of Thames Valley University, the London School of Hospitality, Tourism and Leisure, in particular Elaine O'Sullivan and Liz Plant for allowing me use of university facilities for the photo shoot for this book, and for their overall assistance. Miyoko Imai, Takako Shimogori, Jan Johnson and Teresa Costa for their assistance in preparing food for the photo session. Andrew Milner for proofreading the manuscript.

Craig Willcox, Bradley Willcox and Makoto Suzuki, the co-authors of *The Okinawa Way*, for their permission to reprint their diagrams in this book. Finally, Alexia Chan and Deborah Edwards, and the further education team of Hodder Arnold, for making this book possible, and photographer Sam Bailey for his excellent work.

Introduction

Japanese cuisine has caught on at astonishing speed in major cities across the world. Not just in European and American cities, but also in Mumbai and Auckland, sushi, sashimi and even *kaiseki* are now considered trendy and exotic foods. With rising health awareness everywhere, it was probably only natural that light, fresh and artistically presented food that is conceptually so different from any other cuisine should become popular so quickly – and with enduring effects. Now a growing number of trainee chefs and professionals from diverse culinary backgrounds are taking an interest in this relatively unexplored Asian cookery.

Britain is no exception. Over the three years that I was responsible for designing and teaching Japanese cookery courses at Thames Valley University in London, enthusiasm for Japanese cooking among student chefs as well as professionals increased dramatically. This is what prompted me to write a comprehensive textbook that would be of use both to novices and experienced chefs.

In this book I have outlined the historical development of Japanese cooking, analysed its health benefits, and looked in detail at cooking methods, ingredients and other practical aspects of the culinary art. For the recipes, I have devised easy-to-follow steps for the dishes that are truly authentic, making the instructions as clear and concise as possible. Furthermore, I have devoted a chapter (Chapter 6) to beginners looking for simple recipes that use ingredients readily available in Europe.

I hope this book will give you an insight into the Japanese culture and cuisine and, in so doing, will inspire you to experiment with new cooking methods and ingredients so that your culinary repertoire will be richer and more diverse, and in tune with the global trend.

Lastly, I trust that the growing number of enthusiasts of Japanese cuisine and healthy eating will also find this book a user-friendly companion and rich source of information.

Culture
and Cuisine

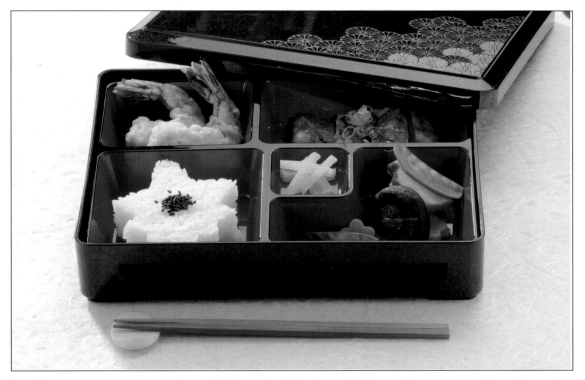

Bento box containing prawn tempura (see p. 128), teriyaki chicken (see p. 74), braised Japanese vegetables, pickles and steamed rice.

Japan is an archipelago extending some 4000 km to the east of the Korean Peninsula, with a climate ranging from subarctic in the north to subtropical at its southern tips. The main island of Honshu, together with the three other major islands of Hokkaido, Shikoku and Kyushu, and over 6800 small islands make up the long, arc-shaped archipelago.

These islands, which cover approximately 375,000 km^2, are much larger than the British isles (220,000 km^2) but, with more than 80 per cent of the land being mountainous and therefore uninhabitable, the Japanese population of over 120 million lives in the plains near the coast, so the usable area is no bigger than Wales. Scarcity of arable land has set limits on cattle farming, but rice is grown throughout the islands. In addition, the nearly 30,000 km of coastline – twice that of Britain – is a rich source of fish and shellfish of immense variety, ranging from blowfish to blue-fin tuna to abalone and lobster. Further, more than 2500 types of seaweed are found in Japanese coastal waters. These geographical factors have undoubtedly shaped the eating habits of Japanese people.

Climatic differences between the extreme northern and the southern ends of the long chain of islands are considerable. However, in most parts, with the exception of Hokkaido and northern Honshu, summer is hot and humid, with the highest temperature exceeding 30 degrees; a brief rainy period precedes a summer that is characterised by typhoons.

In winter, however, Hokkaido and northern Honshu are covered by heavy snow. In Tokyo, where the temperature rarely falls below zero, snow is the exception, but in the ancient capital of Kyoto, despite the summer humidity and heat, winter can be snowy. Most parts of Japan, apart from the subtropical south, have four distinct seasons: between sultry summer and cold, sometimes snowy winter come spring, known for cherry blossom, and autumn, marked by golden leaves. Such dramatic seasonal changes in the natural environment have for centuries been the source of inspiration for traditional Japanese arts such as haiku poetry, the tea ceremony and culinary arts. In formal Japanese cuisine, chefs express seasonal changes of nature by using season-specific ingredients, such as bamboo shoots in spring, wild *ayu* fish in summer or *yuzu* in winter, and by preparing them without altering their inherent flavour or texture. Harmony with the constantly changing natural environment is the essence of traditional Japanese arts, not least cuisine.

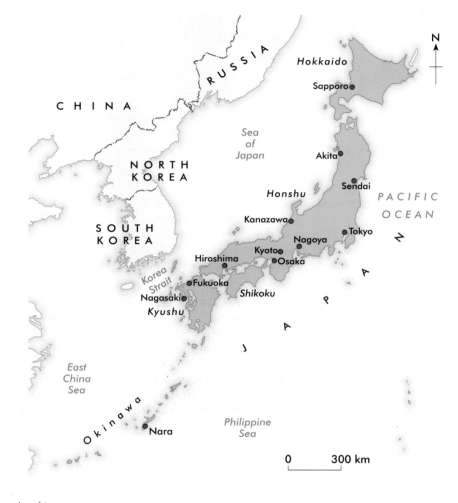

The geography of Japan

chapter 2

HISTORICAL BACKGROUND

Buddhist influence

For centuries, Buddhism has had a strong influence on the Japanese ruling class and their way of life. It was introduced to Japan in the sixth century, and there is unmistakable evidence of this in the Japanese culinary art. The distinctive features – subtle flavour and texture, rich vegetable content and minimalist presentation – that have caught the imagination of culinary enthusiasts worldwide owe their origin to the Buddhist vegetarian cuisine of *shojin-ryori* established in the thirteenth century.

Shojin-ryori, which makes creative use of protein-rich soya beans and a variety of yams, is the invention of vegetarian Zen priests. Minimalist presentation, and imaginative use of pulses and other nutritious vegetables were key features of the Japanese priests' foods. This concept formed the basis of *kaiseki* cuisine, which was served as part of the tea ceremony first patronised by the fifteenth-century Shogun Yoshimasa Ashikaga in Kyoto, the ancient capital of Japan. *Kaiseki* is not vegetarian, though there is an unmistakable Zen overtone, which is part of its unique attraction.

Today, *kaiseki* is often served without the tea ceremony as a sophisticated meal at specialist restaurants in Kyoto and other major cities in Japan – and, to some extent, overseas: it is now recognised worldwide as the finest example of Japanese haute cuisine. Other schools of cuisine, particularly *honzen-ryori*, the banquet cuisine also originating in fifteenth-century Kyoto, have been influenced by *kaiseki*. However, sushi, which emerged as a regional food in the north-east of Kyoto, has a completely different origin.

Soya beans and shojin (Buddhist vegetarian)

Zen priests in thirteenth-century Japan were highly inventive in creating meat substitutes with soya beans. *Ganmodoki*, made of tofu (bean curd) and yam, is probably the best-known example of this. It is popular to this day – available at supermarkets throughout Japan and speciality stores in London. Tofu and its variations, as well as *yuba* (coagulated soya milk) are also frequently used in both *shojin* Buddhist cookery and *kaiseki*.

As strong-flavoured plants such as garlic were forbidden, monastery chefs honed their skills in bringing out the inherent flavour of ingredients

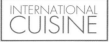
and their unique textural contrasts. This approach to cooking still forms the fundamental principle of Japanese cuisine today.

In both *shojin* and the traditional tea-ceremony *kaiseki*, steamed rice and miso soup are served first, indicating the central role rice plays in the Japanese diet. This remains true today for most meals, formal or informal, and rice is still referred to as the 'main dish'. Moreover, a unique serving rule of *shojin* cuisine is that only lacquer ware is used. This is in contrast to *kaiseki* or the *honzen* banquet cuisine, in which the finest porcelain, as well as lacquer ware, is the essential prop of artistic presentation.

Kaiseki (tea ceremony cuisine)

Historians give credit to the Zen priest Eisai for introducing the tea ceremony to Japan in the early twelfth century after his return from China. It is said that priests drank tea for its supposed healing power, and eventually it became popular with aristocrats and samurai. However, it was to be several centuries before ordinary Japanese people began drinking tea.

From its earliest days, the tea ceremony enjoyed the patronage of Shogun and warlords, and was refined over the centuries under their continuous patronage, which lasted until the mid-nineteenth century when the Shogunate and samurai class were abolished. As the tea ceremony was central to the Shogunate culture, *kaiseki* cuisine, served immediately before the tea, set the standards for the finest culinary arts of the time and this remains true to this day, particularly in Kyoto – home of Japanese haute cuisine. The aesthetic principle of the tea ceremony –

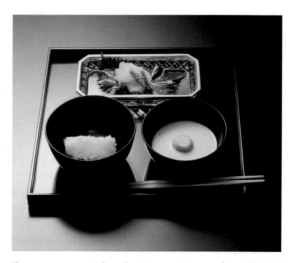

The tea ceremony (photo by Haruomi Nimura, first published in *Tsujitome Tea Ceremony Kaiseki* by Yoshikazu Tsuji, published by Tankosha)

which essentially is harmony with the natural environment – underpins the minimalist presentation of *kaiseki*. As with the tea, the accompanying cuisine is governed by the art of understatement, and dishes are prepared with minimal interference with the inherent flavour, taste and texture of foods. Choice of ingredients, therefore, becomes crucial, particularly when the chef has the added responsibility of expressing on the plate seasonal changes in the environment.

Over the centuries, farmers in Kyoto have cultivated a rich variety of flavoursome and visually attractive vegetables, some of them highly seasonal, in order to meet chefs' special requirements. Kyoto carrots are blood red and its succulent aubergines come in miniature sizes – ideal for minimalist presentation. The Kyoto hills also offer a wide variety of mountain vegetables and herbs rich in natural aroma and texture. While vegetables are crucial to *kaiseki*, fish and poultry are also important, as is (though to a lesser degree) red meat, which is often used thinly sliced and in small quantities.

Modern kaiseki

Some of the top *kaiseki* chefs in Kyoto take the concept of closeness to nature to the extreme and use only wild, local produce – except for vegetables supplied by local farmers. At a celebrated restaurant in central Kyoto, for instance, the chef uses only wild river fish, duck, venison and wild boar meat. He uses also wild herbs or mountain vegetables, picked fresh each morning, and his organic rice is cooked in mountain spring water over a charcoal fire.

At this particular restaurant, a nine-course lunch would consist of a cold plate of vegetables, seaweeds and seafood, followed by a white miso soup, a charcoal barbecued river fish, wild carp *sashimi*, four kinds of vegetables cooked with wild river prawns, charcoal-barbecued duck, another vegetable dish, steamed rice and pickles, and a fruit-based dessert. Each dish – minuscule in size, served in exquisite Kyoto porcelain or lacquer ware and garnished with seasonal wild mountain herbs – is an objet d'art or a miniature flower arrangement. This restaurant, as with many restaurants in Japan today, has broken with traditional practice, and serves rice just before dessert and not at the start of the meal.

In a proper tea ceremony, such a lunch would often be served in a room with a full view of a landscaped garden. *Kaiseki* chefs take pride in offering a wide variety of dishes using a range of the freshest top-quality ingredients that are representative of the particular time of year: it is a highly labour-intensive culinary art. But, as tea masters maintain, *kaiseki* need not be luxurious because it is meant to be an overture to the tea ceremony. At its finest, *kaiseki* is a spiritual experience, as is the tea ceremony.

Serving

Kaiseki is bound by a strict set of rules regarding serving and eating, and the same is true of other styles of formal cuisine developed between the fifteenth and eighteenth centuries: the order in which dishes are served and eaten; the types of ingredients to be used for each course and their cooking methods are laid down. While rules differ from one style of cuisine to another, what they all have in common is that several dishes are served at once on a square lacquer tray. This is true also of the *shojin* Buddhist cuisine. This serving practice persists today in most of Japan, though some restaurants have now adopted the western style of serving one dish at a time.

Depending on the occasion or the style of cuisine, between two and seven trays of dishes are served during a dinner or lunch; the Japanese like to serve to excess when entertaining guests, in order to demonstrate their generosity. This is probably a tradition that persists from the sumptuous *honzen* cuisine, developed for the entertainment of the fifteenth-century samurai. In a typical *honzen* dinner, at least five trays of more than a dozen dishes are served on the understanding that the food on the fourth and fifth trays is for taking home; thus the two final trays are discreetly taken away at an appropriate time and the food neatly packed and handed back to the guests as they leave. This practice of serving to excess and sending guests home with gift-wrapped food for later enjoyment is still very common in Japan today, especially in formal entertainment. However, excessiveness is clearly contrary to the Zen principle and this custom does not apply to *kaiseki*.

Sushi

Sushi initially came about as a way of preserving fish in north-east Kyoto. By first curing fish in salt, then washing the salt away before smothering the fish with rice for fermentation in its lactic acid, fifteenth-century Japanese turned the most perishable food into a preserve that would keep for months. At this time 'sushi' was not served on rice.

Following the introduction of rice vinegar in the mid-seventeenth century, vinegared rice (or sushi rice), containing vinegar and salt, came into being. Then eventually the rice was combined with vinegar-marinated fish to become sushi, as we know it today. *Bo-zushi* (stick sushi), which is a long rectangular-shaped sushi made of a whole fish fillet, is one of the earliest forms of sushi from the period, and mackerel *bo-zushi* is still a Kyoto staple today. Subsequently, *oshi-zushi* (pressed sushi) and *hako-zushi* (box sushi) were developed in Kyoto and Osaka, followed by *chirashi-zushi* (scattered sushi). *Maki-zushi* (rolled sushi) as well as *inari-zushi* (vegetarian sushi made with *age* – deep-fried tofu)   also emerged.

The bite-size *nigiri-zushi*, or hand-formed sushi, was a later invention, developed as the fast food of working men in early nineteenth-century

Tokyo (or Edo as it was known then), which by then had outgrown Osaka and Kyoto as the biggest town in Japan under the Tokugawa Shogunate. An influx of craftsmen and artisans from the countryside created a demand for fast food, and *nigiri-zushi* – a variety that uses raw, uncured fish and requires minimum preparation – emerged. Sushi stalls sprouted, along with stalls for other types of fast food such as soba, or buckwheat noodles (see p. 63). As fish was plentiful in Tokyo Bay at the time, prices were low. Several decades later, following the great earthquake of 1923 that devastated Tokyo, surviving sushi chefs fled to the countryside. In this way, *nigiri-zushi* spread to other parts of Japan.

Nigiri-zushi dominance

A nationwide push for *nigiri-zushi* in preference to Kyoto- and Osaka-style sushi, came from an unexpected source, namely the Allied occupation authorities following the end of the Second World War. Faced with a severe food shortage, the authorities issued a decree allowing Japanese people to exchange a cup of uncooked rice for ten pieces of *nigiri-zushi*. Unaware of other forms of sushi, the Allied authorities inadvertently excluded them all. As a result, many sushi shops stopped serving traditional sushi, and the damage had a lasting effect. In Tokyo and elsewhere *nigiri-zushi* is the most popular form of sushi, though in Osaka and Kyoto local sushi still has a huge following – particularly because it keeps longer and goes with other foods. Kyoto-style sushi is often served in the tea ceremony *kaiseki*, but never *nigiri-zushi*. *Nigiri-zushi* tastes best as soon as it is formed and is not intended for preserving, which was the original intention of sushi.

Kyoto- and Osaka-style sushi, however, tend to be heavy on rice. There are restaurants specialising in *chirashi-zushi*, for instance, but this type of sushi, along with rolled sushi, can easily be made at home. As the price of fish, especially of sushi quality, continues to escalate, creative *nigiri-zushi*, using cooked vegetables, pickles or even a miniature steak, is catching on. California roll, made with crab-sticks, avocado and mayonnaise is a US West Coast invention that has become popular across the world. Sushi allows infinite scope for creativity.

Regional cooking

We have looked at haute cuisine in detail mainly because *kaiseki* and its modern variations are at the forefront of Japanese cuisine today, internationally and domestically. But being composed of a geographically diverse group of islands, Japan offers a rich variety of regional cooking, which is enjoyed with minimum ceremony. In fact, wherever there is a great fishing port there is a distinct regional food because the Japanese love fish. For instance, Shimonoseki, in south-west Japan, is well known for poisonous blowfish and its food culture based on this fish, which has for centuries been a delicacy in Japan. (Poisonous veins are completely

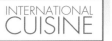
removed and the flesh is eaten as a special one-pot dish or *sashimi*.) Unique to Akita, northern Honshu, is *kiri-tanpo*, a one-pot dish of chicken, vegetables and tofu in chicken stock that is eaten with grilled rice sticks.

Meat and sukiyaki

Meat consumption is still small-scale in Japan compared with Europe and the United States, but *sukiyaki* (see p. 165 for the recipe), a one-pot dish of thinly sliced beef, vegetables and tofu cooked in a seasoned liquid, remains a classic Japanese beef dish to this day. Eating meat was banned by a seventh-century emperor (apparently to protect wild horses) and, although the ban was subsequently lifted, the tradition had become so firmly established that it was to be more than 1000 years before the Meiji Emperor reintroduced meat to the Japanese diet in the early nineteenth century. *Sukiyaki* was one of the first meat dishes developed at the time, as Japan opened its doors to the West and its culinary influences. Decades later, *shabu-shabu* (see p. 161 for the recipe), another one-pot dish of paper-thin beef and vegetables eaten with sesame sauce or *ponzu* (soy and citrus sauce, see p. 43), was invented. A variety of braised or grilled meat dishes has also emerged, some of which have been refined for *kaiseki*.

Japanese cuisine has evolved over the centuries, but its fundamental structure and principles have remained intact, particularly in formal cuisine. Today, a cross-section of Japanese and western culinary enthusiasts dine at *kaiseki* restaurants, attracted by the atmospheric setting and artistic presentation as much as by the food they offer. Japanese cuisine at its finest embraces Zen and the sophisticated arts of Shogunate Kyoto.

THE HEALTH BENEFITS OF JAPANESE FOOD

chapter 3

Longevity

The Japanese are the longest-living people in the world, according to the World Health Organization (WHO). Its statistics show that Japan holds top place with an average life expectancy of 82 years, while Britain ranks eighteenth with 78 years and the United States twentieth with 77 years. Gerontologists, cardiologists and geriatricians maintain that it is Japanese people's eating habits and their overall lifestyle – and not their genes – that are the primary reasons for their outstanding health. Health benefit is clearly one of the biggest reasons for the phenomenal popularity of Japanese food today.

Hormone-induced cancer and chronic diseases

Long life expectancy, according to medical experts, is a result of avoiding chronic diseases such as cancer, diabetes, stroke and cardiovascular disease. Studies show that the rates of breast cancer and prostate cancer, which are among the biggest killers in the UK and USA, are dramatically lower in Japan. The same is true of other hormone-dependent cancers, such as those of the ovary or colon.

Further, most Japanese women have a natural menopause, hormone replacement treatment (HRT) being extremely rare. Indeed, research indicates that fewer Japanese women suffer from oestrogen deficiency than do women in Europe or the United States. And, within Japan, women in Okinawa – a group of islands in the southernmost part of Japan, where life expectancy far exceeds the national average – suffer least from hormone deficiency. Canadian and Japanese research scientists who specialise in studying the longevity of Okinawans point to their eating habits, which are characterised by high consumption of tofu, bean curd (see p. 49) and other soya bean products rich in the plant oestrogens known as flavonoids. Tofu is eaten throughout Japan – traditionally in miso soup or on its own with soy sauce and condiments – but Okinawan Japanese consume it in much larger quantities. Their regional tofu, made with fresh sea water, is firmer so is often stir-fried with vegetables, and sometimes with meat. Researchers say that the

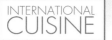

tofu-rich diet is what primarily gives Okinawan Japanese a few extra years of robust health compared with mainland Japanese – and the rest of the world.[1]

Tofu and soya bean products

Soya beans are eaten in a variety of ways in Japan, tofu being only one of them. They are a complete protein containing cholesterol-free fat, notably omega-3. Moreover, there are scientific studies that underscore the soya bean's ability to fight heart diseases and hormone-dependent cancers, such as those of the breast and prostate. A clinical trial at the University of Texas showed that women who ate a soy-fortified diet for one month saw their blood oestrogen (a risk factor for breast cancer) fall by 20 per cent.[2] Scientists maintain that firm tofu is particularly high in flavonoid content, compared with the softer silken kind. Flavonoids (weak plant oestrogens) provide a mild oestrogen-like effect post-menopausally; research shows strong oestrogen withdrawal effects such as hot flushes are reduced without increasing cancer risks.

Cardiovascular diseases are also sharply lower in Japan where, historically, they have never been a major cause of death. A number of scientists consider that the beneficial effects of a soya bean-rich diet, as well as the low cholesterol and calorie content of traditional Japanese foods, are the main reasons for this phenomenon.

Fewer calories – low cholesterol

The total calorie content of a typical Japanese meal is estimated at approximately 1800, which is considerably lower than the approximate 2500 calories of an average western meal. With fish, and tofu and its variations being the main source of protein, and meat eaten only in small quantities in Japan, such a calorie difference is not surprising. The Japanese eat a great many low-calorie vegetable dishes as well as steamed rice – the main source of carbohydrates in Japan (and lower in calories than white bread). Moreover, virtually fat-free cooking methods – grilling, steaming or simmering – also minimise calorie content. *Tonkatsu* and *tempura* – two well-known deep-fried dishes – were originally western concepts.

Theoretically, therefore, eating traditionally Japanese foods should make dieting unnecessary, allowing you to eat to your heart's content without fear of weight gain, as long as the bulk of the food comes from the bottom rung of the caloric density pyramid pictured opposite.

1. Willcox, B., Willcox, C. and Suzuki, M. (2001) *The Okinawa Way*. Mermaid Books.
2. Lu, L.J. and Anderson, M. (2001) Effects of an isoflavone-free soy diet on ovarian hormones in premenopausal women, *Journal of Clinical Endocrinology & Metabolism* 86 (7), 3045–52.

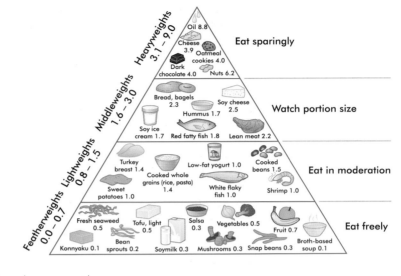

Caloric density pyramid

This calorie pyramid shows that Japanese foods are almost entirely free of 'heavyweights', the majority being 'featherweights', which are predominantly antioxidant-rich vegetables, seaweed, tofu and fruits.

The diagram below compares the calorie density of a cheeseburger with that of a light Okinawan Japanese meal of stir-fried vegetables, rice and miso soup. Both meals contain 280 calories but the Japanese meal is

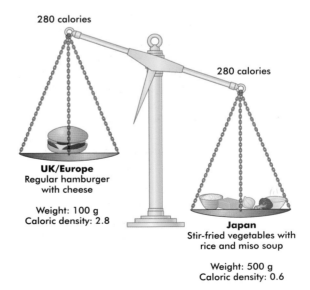

Calorie density comparison: cheeseburger vs light Okinawan meal

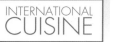

bulkier, weighing five times more than the cheeseburger; hence it is more filling despite having the same number of calories. Japanese elders who have adhered to a traditional diet are slim: an overweight centenarian is a contradiction in terms.

There is now overwhelming evidence to show that calorie restriction extends lifespan. Controlled experiments with animals have demonstrated conclusively that nutritiously dense and low-calorie feeds cause animals to live up to 30 per cent longer, according to research scientists specialising in longevity.[3] Moreover, the low-calorie studies of the Gerontology Research Center at the National Institute on Aging in Maryland, in the United States, show that primates on a low-calorie diet demonstrated health improvements such as improved blood sugar control, youthful appearance, leaner bodies, and increased mental sharpness.

However, as these animal studies have highlighted, high nutritious density is vital in calorie-restricted diets, which means they should be rich in the antioxidants that neutralise the cell-damaging free radicals released during metabolism (see below). The best sources of antioxidants, scientists emphasise, are vegetables, seaweed, fruit, grains and pulses such as soya beans.

Antioxidants

Antioxidants have aroused strong interest among health experts and sports scientists alike. Vitamins E and C, beta-carotene and selenium are the major substances with antioxidant functions that prevent cell-damaging oxidation when the human body converts foods into energy – the process known as metabolising. The free radicals, or oxidants that are unstable molecules created during metabolising, are responsible for oxidation; antioxidants mop up these substances. Your body has natural defences, including its own antioxidants, but medical experts recommend loading up on them from food sources, as DNA and important cellular constituents are constantly exposed to free radicals. Besides, as research by the US National Institute on Aging has shown, less cellular damage also means less damage to collagen in the skin, which means fewer wrinkles!

However, scientists do not recommend taking antioxidant supplements, advising people instead to source this anti-ageing substance from dietary sources. The recommendation of the American Institute for Cancer Research is five servings of fruit and vegetables a day, but studies show that the Japanese who enjoy robust health into their nineties – and beyond – eat, on average, seven servings a day.[4]

---

3. Willcox, Willcox and Suzuki, *Okinawa Way*.
4. Willcox, Willcox and Suzuki, *Okinawa Way*.

Antioxidant-rich foods

Nearly all antioxidant-rich foods – vegetables, seaweed, grains and fruit – come from the bottom rung of the caloric density pyramid (see diagram, p. 13). This means that, in theory, you can eat these foods until you are stuffed – and be healthier and slimmer for it! And as you will see in the later chapters, there are hundreds of ways of making mouth-watering dishes using these healthy ingredients. Establishing an eating habit based on these power foods, it seems, is the key to health and longevity – and a slim and youthful body. We looked at soya beans earlier in this chapter; the following are other examples of power foods and their health benefits.

Examples of power foods

Konnyaku (devil's tongue jelly)

Konnyaku, made from the yam starch known as devil's tongue (see p. 67), has been a popular food in Japan and China for centuries. Despite having a calorie rating of zero, *konnyaku* is filling because it is composed almost entirely of water and soluble plant fibre known as glucomannan. For this reason, it has long been considered a highly effective weapon in the battle for weight control. However, clinical trials have also shown that this soluble fibre is effective in the treatment of high cholesterol and constipation, and a beneficial adjunct for treatment of Type II (adult-onset) diabetes.[5]

Fermented foods

The health benefits of fermented foods are recognised throughout the world. Research has shown that fermentation can inhibit pathogenic bacteria, enhance digestive power, suppress toxins and anti-nutritive substance and, in the case of soya beans, boost its flavonoid content. The traditional Japanese diet is rich in fermented products such as soy sauce, *sake*, *mirin*, miso and *natto* (p. 51).

Natto is fermented cooked soya beans. These have been eaten in Japan for over 1000 years. (Fermentation is aided by beneficial bacteria Bacillus *natto*.) Clinical trials have shown that the nattokinase enzyme in *natto* dissolves the blood clots that can lead to heart attack, stroke and senility.[6]

---

5. Department of Nutritional Sciences (2001) St Michael's Hospital, Faculty of Medicine, University of Toronto, Ontario, Canada (and others).
6. Dr Hiroyuki Sumi, (1980) Research paper, Chicago University Medical School; 1995 clinical trials at Miyazaki Medical College and Kurashiki University of Science and Arts, Japan.

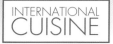

Seaweed (*konbu* or kelp, *nori*, *hijiki* and *wakame*)

Seaweed, which comes in more than 5000 varieties, provides a rich supply of many essential nutrients, including protein, calcium, zinc and iodine. It is a champion of nutritiously dense and low-calorie food: half a cup of kelp contains only 50 calories but provides 2 grams of protein, 20 mg of magnesium, as well as iron and calcium, analysis shows. Moreover, lignans, the cancer-fighting phytoestrogens (plant oestrogens), have been found in high quantity in seaweed, predominantly in kelp. *Nori*, used in sushi rolls, is exceptionally high in protein and even lower in calories than kelp.

The only drawback of seaweed is its sodium content. Half a cup of *wakame* contains approximately 900 mg of sodium, 15 per cent of the 6 gm daily limit recommended by nutritionists. Kelp and laver have less sodium, however, containing 250 mg and 6 mg respectively on average in half a cup. Scientists advise against taking seaweed supplements because of a possible overload of iron and other side effects. It is best to enjoy seaweed as food.

Omega-3-rich fish

Not all fats are bad, medical experts emphasise. Much has been written about the health benefits of polyunsaturated fats, namely omega-3 and omega-6: they help prevent heart disease and other chronic diseases by lowering bad cholesterol (LDL) while maintaining healthy cholesterol (HDL). A major source of this type of fat is dark-fleshed fish such as mackerel, tuna, sardine and salmon, which are eaten widely in Japan. The low rate of heart disease among the Japanese validates this point. Studies show that the Inuit, whose diet is mostly fish and other marine animals, also have a low rate of heart disease. These dark-fleshed fish have, on average, a 12 per cent fat content compared with swordfish and bonito tuna, which have roughly 6 per cent, and white-fleshed fish such as sea bream, cod, haddock and halibut, which have a less than 2.5 per cent fat content. At 12 per cent, the fat content of fatty fish is still lower than that of lean beef, and helps keep arteries clean by reducing harmful cholesterol. Cod liver oil is omega-3 fat. In cod, oil is concentrated in the liver, whereas in the darker-fleshed fish, fat is spread throughout the fish, giving it a darker colour and stronger flavour. Dried bonito, whose shavings form the basis of Japanese soup stock, or *dashi*, is also a source of omega-3.

Shiitake

This large, flat and dark brown mushroom, available at supermarkets throughout the UK, is rich in vitamin D. It is an ideal ingredient for any healthy, low-fat, low-calorie dish.

Adzuki

The tiny, dark-red adzuki beans that have been grown in Asia for centuries are, like most beans, rich in soluble fibre, which helps to eliminate cholesterol. Extremely popular across Asia, they are cooked with sugar to make a sweet, red bean paste for pastry fillings or desserts. High in protein but low in calories, adzuki beans provide a healthy alternative to animal protein: one cup of cooked adzuki beans contain fewer than 230 calories, and they are an excellent source of potassium, iron, magnesium, copper, zinc and vitamin B3.

Sodium

High sodium content has long been considered a drawback in the Japanese diet. Stroke used to be the biggest killer in Japan because of the high salt intake. However, overall salt intake, though still higher on average than that in Britain or the United States, has dropped considerably as a result of persistent nationwide campaigns in the media and by health authorities. In addition, improved refrigeration facilities mean that it is no longer necessary to use salt as a preservative in dried fish, miso and many other products. Special low-sodium miso and soy sauce are available for those who need to limit their sodium intake.

The modern diet and its devastating effect

We have looked at the health benefits of the traditional Japanese diet, which research scientists and physicians have concluded is one of the key factors behind the world's longest life expectancy. However, these scientists also predict that the younger generation of Japanese, who have adopted a fast-food culture and higher fat-content diets, are likely to face shorter life expectancy as obesity, diabetes and cardiovascular risk factors have increased. Recent studies show that while a 65-year-old Japanese male is expected to live to 82.5, a 20 year old is likely to live only to 78.3.[7] However, traditional eating habits are belatedly making a comeback among young, weight-conscious Japanese, which is a sign that they, like the rest of the world, are waking up to their health benefits.

7. Willcox, C.D. (2005) Okinawa longevity: where do we go from here? *Nutrition & Dietetics* 8(1).

The traditional structure of a Japanese meal is 'one soup three dishes' (1 汁 3 菜) plus a bowl of rice and pickles. The three dishes are typically a grilled dish and two supplementary dishes of smaller portions. Unlike western meals, preparation methods rather than ingredients, determine the choice of the three dishes. Variety and harmony are two guiding principles of menu planning; seasonal quality is third. Another distinctive characteristic of a Japanese meal is that, as mentioned earlier, all dishes are traditionally placed on a lacquer tray and served to each individual. In big meals there could be two or three trays, each comprising three or more dishes, but conventionally all trays are presented simultaneously, the exception being in the tea ceremony, when dishes are served in several 'courses'.

As a result, not all dishes are expected to be served piping hot, except for the soup and rice, but their harmony when designing a menu becomes crucial, as they are all eaten together.

The grilled dish could be fish, poultry or even red meat. One of the supplementary items is usually a vegetable dish, and the other could be a tofu dish, pulses or seaweed. *Sashimi* is served in addition to the other three when the occasion demands it.

An example of a 'one soup three dishes' meal would be grilled chicken, a tofu dish and a vegetable in dressing, to which *sashimi* could be added as a special treat – to liven up the occasion.

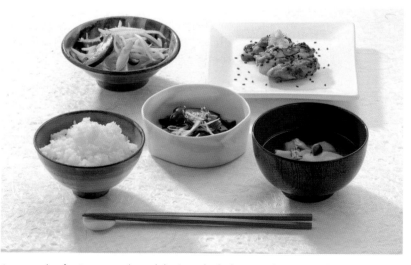

An example of a 'one soup three dishes' meal: chicken teriyaki set menu (see p. 74)

Tools and Ingredients

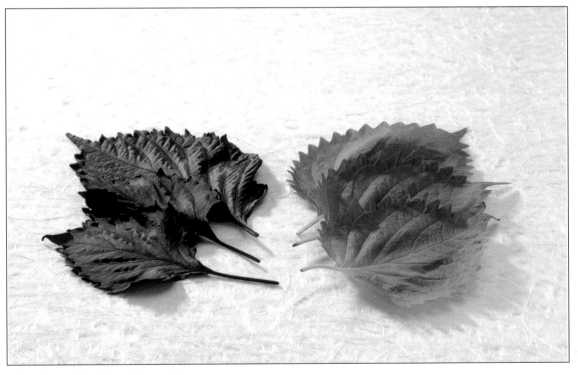

Red and green shiso leaves (see p. 59)

chapter 5

BASIC KITCHEN TOOLS

Knives

Sharp knives with the right type of blade are crucial to Japanese cookery, especially for formal cuisine. More cutting and slicing take place in Japanese cooking than in European cooking. Ingredients have to be cut into bite-size pieces so that they can be eaten with chopsticks, but this has to be done skilfully, especially when slicing *sashimi*, in order to perfect the artistic presentation and preserve the textural quality. Knives and cutting techniques, therefore, are immensely important. Chefs are often obsessive about their tools. As the saying goes, 'knives are the soul of Japanese chefs'.

Professional knives are made of forged or laminated steel for sharpness and strength. Many of these blades have a cutting edge on one side only, which chefs sharpen daily on a fine-grained whetstone. Three principal knives are illustrated below.

Vegetable knife (nakiri-bocho)

This is a vegetable-cutting knife, and is used solely for vegetable preparation. The sharp, long (about 18 cm) and rectangular blade peels, slices and chops vegetables with efficiency and speed. A *nakiri-bocho* has a cutting edge on both sides of the blade, as do western knives, which gives a clean edge to vegetables. This knife is light and should be well balanced.

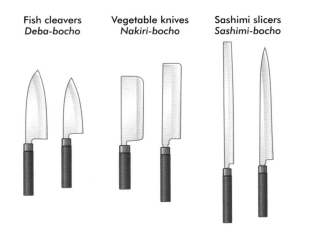

Fish cleavers
Deba-bocho   Vegetable knives
Nakiri-bocho   Sashimi slicers
Sashimi-bocho

The three principle knives used in Japanese cookery (L–R): fish cleavers (*deba-bocho*), vegetable knives (*nakiri-bocho*) and *sashimi* slicers (*sashimi-bocho*)

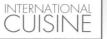

Fish cleavers (deba-bocho)

This knife has a sharp, heavy and pointed blade and is an efficient tool for gutting, boning or filleting fish. The blade comes in a variety of lengths, between 10 cm and 30 cm. The sharp point makes gutting easier, and its sharp and weighty blade cuts through a thick fish bone or head in a single stroke. Made of carbon steel, there is little danger of chipping. This knife, which has a cutting edge on one side of the blade, is also useful for cutting poultry – through the bone – or meat.

Sashimi knife (sashimi-bocho)

This is a knife specifically designed for slicing filleted fish for *sashimi*. The long – about 20 cm to 40 cm – and narrow, sharp blade produces the slices with clean edges that are crucial for *sashimi*. There are two types of *sashimi* knife – one with a sharp point and one with a blunt top. They are both equally efficient. This knife has a cutting edge on one side only.

Useful tools for Japanese cookery

Sushi rice cooling tub (sushi-oke, hangiri)

This is a shallow, flat-bottomed wooden bowl for rapidly mixing vinegar into steamed rice, without crushing its grains. The large wooden tub absorbs the moisture of the rice and helps to cool it quickly, preventing it getting soggy. Select a tub that has a smooth surface and a hint of cedar wood aroma. Soak it in water for half an hour before use in order to make the wood more absorbent.

Rice paddle (shamoji)

This paddle, which looks like a curved spatula, is an instrument for mixing rice without crushing its grains. Traditionally it is made of wood, but now there are non-stick plastic kinds, which are extremely efficient.

Graters (oroshi-gane)

A Japanese grater, fitted with sharp pointed spikes, is a must in Japanese cooking. These sharp spikes are designed for finely grating fibrous vegetables such as ginger and *daikon* radish (mooli). European graters are not sharp enough for this purpose. Large graters designed for *daikon* radish give coarser results than the smaller ones for ginger or *wasabi*. They come in strong plastic or metal.

Vegetable slicers

Japanese slicers with sharp metal or ceramic blades are useful for making paper-thin slices of crunchy vegetables. Ultra-thin slices of celery or cucumber lend themselves well to Japanese salads and garnishes. Ceramic blades are very efficient and easier to clean than metal ones.

Chopsticks (hashi)

Japanese chopsticks are pointed and shorter than the Chinese kind, but long cooking chopsticks (about 40 cm in length) are useful aids in the kitchen for stirring, turning over and picking up delicate foods. Usually made of bamboo, there are metal-tipped ones for deep-frying.

Vegetable cutters (yasai-gata)

These metal cutters, which resemble biscuit cutters, are useful for cutting vegetables into regular shapes or decorative pieces. Carrot slices cut into cherry blossoms or maple leaves, for instance, make excellent garnishes. These cutters are sold individually or as a set.

Fan (uchiwa)

A large fan is useful for rapidly cooling down sushi rice in the tub. Rice is continuously fanned until it cools to room temperature, ready for sushi.

Square omelette pan (maki-yaki nabe)

This shallow rectangular pan is an essential instrument for making rolled omelettes. It enables you to fry and roll omelettes of uniform thickness into a neat cylinder. Professional chefs use tin-coated copper pans but non-stick pans are also available.

Bamboo sushi mat (maki-su)

This square bamboo mat is the tool for forming and pressing rolled sushi (*maki-zushi*) and rolled omelettes into cylindrical shapes. Resembling a miniature bamboo blind, it is made of thin bamboo slats held together by strong cotton string. The mat is typically a 25 cm square. It must be washed and dried thoroughly after use.

Rice cooker

Most Japanese use an electric rice cooker, which makes perfect rice. These are inexpensive and available in Britain.

Oil skimmer (ami jakushi)

This scoop made of fine metal mesh is an efficient tool for skimming bits of batter from cooking oil, and keeping the oil clean. It is an essential aid when making *tempura*.

Deep-frying pot (agemono-nabe)

Pots used for deep-frying in Japanese cookery should be deep and heavy, preferably cast-iron, as they best maintain a large quantity of oil at a high temperature.

Oil draining rack and tray

This is a shallow rectangular pan fitted with a rack for draining off oil. Deep-fried foods are placed on the rack to drain before they are arranged on individual serving plates covered with folded absorbent paper.

Cooking methods

Cooking takes place on the stove in Japan. The oven was never developed in the long history of Japanese cooking; charcoal barbecuing is the most traditional method and is still used in many professional kitchens today. The following sections describe the five principal methods of Japanese cookery.

Simmering

Gentle boiling over a low, constant heat is a classic cooking method in Japan. The key to successful simmering is minimal heat: heat so low that there is hardly any movement on the surface of the food being cooked. Almost any food is suitable for simmering, including root vegetables, tofu, sliced meat and even whole fish, and they are cooked in a seasoned *dashi* stock (see the recipe on p. 119 for simmered *daikon* radish). For professional results, however, a drop-in lid (*otoshi-buta*) is essential (as shown in the picture below). This small lid drops on to the foods inside a saucepan and holds them in place as they slowly cook. A small plate can be used instead of a drop-in lid as long as it is light enough not to crush the foods. This inner lid also speeds up cooking by trapping heat underneath it.

To make a successful simmered dish, bear in mind the following key points.

- The drop-in lid (see illustration) should be at least 2.5 cm smaller in diameter than the saucepan.

- When adding seasonings to a stock, sugar should always go in first. Salt, soy sauce and other seasonings should go in only after the sugar has been absorbed as salt blocks the absorption of sugar.

- Each ingredient should be cut into pieces of the same size so that everything cooks at the same rate. Uniformity in the size and shape of each ingredient is also an advantage in presentation.

Grilling and barbecuing

Direction of heat source distinguishes grilling from barbecuing: in the former, heat is applied

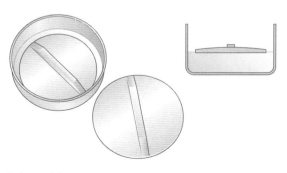

A drop-in lid

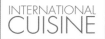

from above and, in the latter, from below. In Japanese cuisine, charcoal barbecuing is a classic method, and considered the ideal means of cooking fish. In Japan, many professional kitchens are equipped with charcoal facilities, though gas barbecuing is becoming increasingly common. Aside from fish, poultry and vegetables may also be served barbecued using either gas or charcoal, *yakitori* (see p. 149 for recipe) being one of the best-known examples. Grilled or barbecued fish or poultry should be moist and succulent inside but crisp and brown – not burnt – on the outside. When barbecuing a whole fish, Japanese chefs often use what is known as the 'wave skewering' technique, which leaves the fish looking as if it is actively 'swimming upstream' on the plate.

Here are some key points to bear in mind when grilling or barbecuing.

- Temperature control is vital for successful results.
- Grill under high heat and adjust the heat's distance from the food in order to control temperature.
- When grilling a whole fish, start with the side that will be presented to the diner.
- When grilling a filleted fish, start with the flesh side, not the skin.
- Turn the skewers a few times during grilling so that they can be extracted easily.

Shallow-frying and stir-frying

Frying in a shallow layer of oil is relatively new to Japanese cookery, barbecuing and simmering being the more traditional methods. However, today this technique is applied in a variety of ways, to meat as well as vegetables. Sliced meat is often pan-fried – or seared in the minimum amount of oil – in order to 'seal in' its flavour (see p. 160 for a recipe for pork loin with ginger-flavoured soy sauce). Vegetables are cut into small pieces and stir-fried – or fried rapidly while being tossed frequently to obtain even cooking and colouring – either on their own or with meat.

Bear in mind the following key points when shallow- or stir-frying.

- When stir-frying, cut each ingredient into pieces of a uniform size so that they all cook at the same rate and quickly.
- Fry those ingredients that require the longest cooking time first, and gradually add the others in order of required cooking time.
- A frequent and rapid tossing action is necessary when stir-frying in order to minimise the amount of oil required. This is important as it prevents food getting too oily.

Deep-frying

This is not a cooking method indigenous to Japan, having been introduced into the country first by the Chinese and later by Europeans.

Deep-frying is nevertheless a speedy means of cooking by submerging food in oil that has been heated to approximately 160–180°C. For a light and crispy result, oil must be hot enough to seal the outside surface of the food, while leaving the inside moist and succulent. The appropriate temperature of oil varies according to the type of food being fried and its size. The Japanese have refined the deep-frying technique for *tempura* (see p. 128 for recipe) to an art form. The best *tempura* dishes are extremely light because the ingredients, coated in feather-light batter, have been fried very swiftly in a pool of high-temperature vegetable oil. (In Japan, each *tempura* specialist has his/her own unique blend of oil.) The amount of high-quality oil and the frying skills required mean that, in reality, top-quality *tempura* can be eaten only at a specialist restaurant where a chef fries in front of customers seated at a counter. In addition to those used with *tempura*, other deep-frying techniques are frequently used in Japanese cooking – namely, frying foods with no coating (*su-age*) or lightly dusted with flour (*kara-age*). Deep-fried marinated chicken (see p. 146) is a popular *kara-age* dish. Deep-fried food, be it *tempura*, *su-age* or *kara-age*, should be light and golden yellow, crunchy on the outside and moist inside.

Here are a few key points to bear in mind when deep-frying.

- Clean, good-quality vegetable oil must be used, and in sufficient quantity.
- Fill the fryer about 60 per cent full with oil.
- The temperature of the oil must be kept constant throughout frying.
- Fry vegetables first, before fish or meat.
- Remove crumbs constantly in order to keep the oil clean.
- Foods should be cut to a manageable size to permit speedy cooking.
- Do not fry too many pieces at once.
- Filter the oil using absorbent paper immediately after frying.

Steaming

This is a method of cooking food that uses the vapour from boiling water kept 'trapped' within a vessel. Cooked in this way, food retains its moisture – and therefore its flavour – and any risk of burning is minimised. For these reasons, steaming is best suited to cooking foods that have a delicate texture and/or flavour, such as fish, seafood, chicken and savoury custard cup (see recipe on p. 125). However, in order to enhance their inherent flavour some ingredients are marinated prior to steaming. Another advantage of steaming is that it allows food to retain its shape and appearance better than some other cooking methods. Moreover, as moisture loss is minimised, any nutrients present are better preserved.

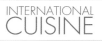
Bear in mind the following key points when steaming.

- Wait until vapour begins to rise before placing food in the steamer.

- Timing is critical in steaming. Do not over-steam.

- Steaming is appropriate only for fresh and good-quality ingredients as this cooking technique relies almost entirely on their inherent flavour and taste. If the food is tasteless to start with, select another method.

Cutting techniques

Japanese cuisine is known for its artistic presentation. In formal cuisine in particular, visual effects are considered almost as important as the taste of a dish. Cutting fresh ingredients with precision into the required shapes and sizes is essential for the visual success of a dish. Moreover, precise cutting is equally important to achieve the desired textural effects in food – an important element of Japanese cuisine. The following sections look at some of the most frequently used cutting techniques.

Standard vegetable cuts

Root vegetables, primarily *daikon* radishes (mooli) and carrots, are cut into the shapes illustrated below.

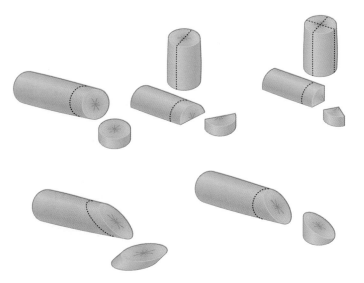

Carrot cuts: rounds; half-rounds; quarters; diagonals; rolling cut; the latter is used with root vegetables, such as carrots, *daikon* radishes, burdock and bamboo shoots, which are cut in this way to give them a bigger surface area

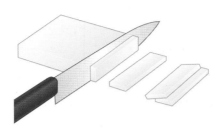

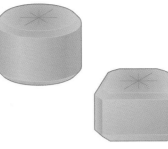

Rectangles: this is an attractive cut for soups and salads; it is most often used with root vegetables and stem vegetables such as celery

Bevelling: this technique is used with root vegetables or tubers to keep their shapes intact when simmered

Decorative cuts

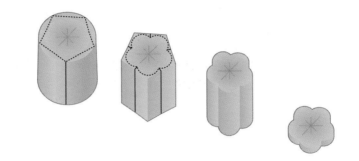

Carrots and radish flowers: this cut is often used for simmered dishes, for visual effect

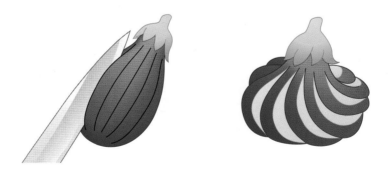

Aubergine whisk: this special cut is used in deep-fried aubergine dishes

29

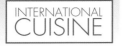

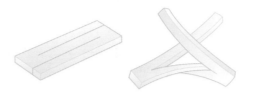

Citrus rind pine needle: *yuzu* (a tangerine-sized
citrus fruit) is cut in this way for garnishing clear
soups; it works well with lemon too – cut rind into a
1 cm–wide rectangle and make a 2–3 mm incision
from opposite ends; open it up to make it stand

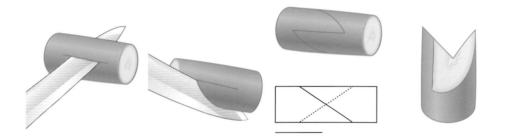

Vegetable peaks: these peaks make an attractive garnish for grilled dishes

Prawns: skewer with a cocktail stick to
prevent the prawn curling when cooked

Gutting techniques
Gutting through the gills

This is a conventional way of gutting a small fish that leaves the cavity intact so that the fish can be served whole.

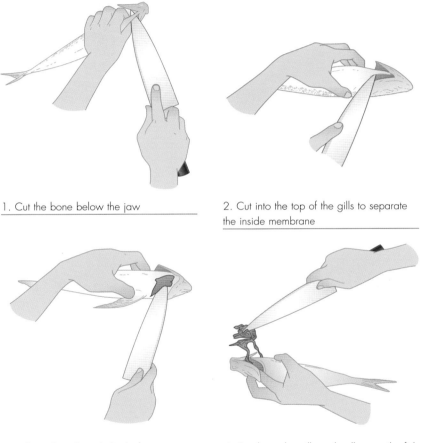

1. Cut the bone below the jaw

2. Cut into the top of the gills to separate the inside membrane

3. Pull out the gills with the knife tip

4. Pin down the gills and pull away the fish

Removing the guts through the mouth (tsubo-nuki)

The fish can be gutted in this way only if it is extremely fresh.

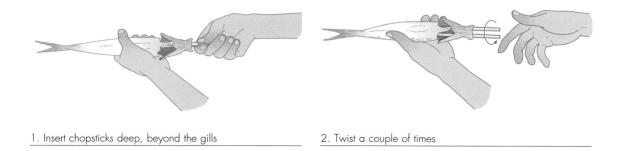

1. Insert chopsticks deep, beyond the gills

2. Twist a couple of times

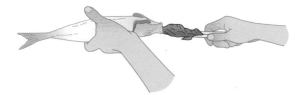

3. Slowly pull out the guts together with the gills

Round fish filleting technique

Three-piece filleting

This is the traditional Japanese way of filleting a fish. Make sure that all the scales have been removed.

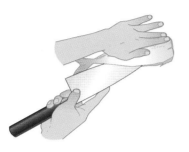

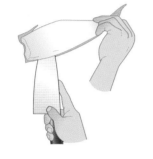

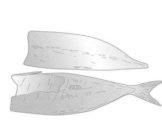

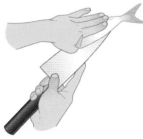

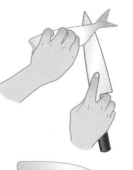

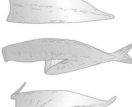

Following the steps illustrated here, one boneless fillet is cut from each side of the fish and the skeleton is left as a third piece

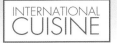
Flat fish filleting technique

Five-piece filleting

This technique, which is used only with flat fish, is also used by western chefs.

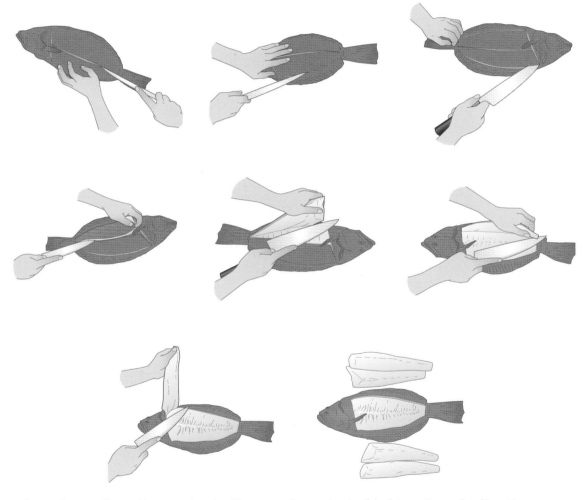

Following the steps illustrated here, two boneless fillets are cut from each side of the fish, resulting in four fillets. The remaining carcass makes a fifth piece

Filleting for *sashimi*

First, fillet the fish using the three-piece filleting technique (see p. 33), then prepare it for *sashimi* following the steps illustrated below.

1st fillet

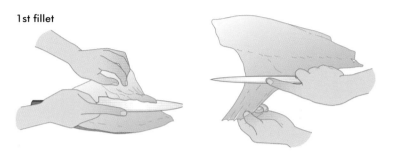

Take a fillet and remove the bones that line the visceral cavity

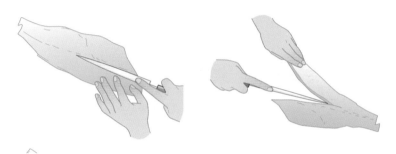

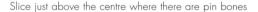

Slice just above the centre where there are pin bones

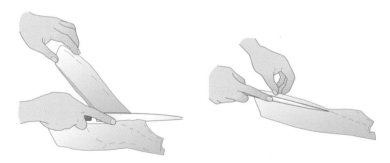

Cut as far as where the fillet narrows, then cut up at an angle to form two pieces of equal width

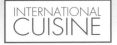

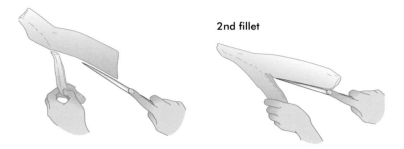

2nd fillet

Cut along the centre line of the other piece to remove the pin bone strip

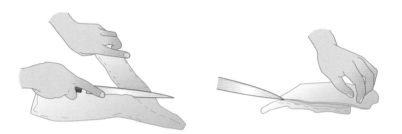

For the second fillet, repeat the steps illustrated here

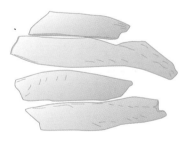

Four fillets, ready for *sashimi*

Sashimi slicing technique

There are a number of *sashimi* slicing techniques, but the 'rectangular technique' applicable to any type of fish, including tuna and snapper, is illustrated below. A *sashimi* knife (see p. 21) is a must.

1. Place the fillet on a chopping board with the skinned side up and the belly side facing you.

2. Place your left hand lightly on the fillet. Hold the knife so that the tip of the blade is leaning slightly to the left.

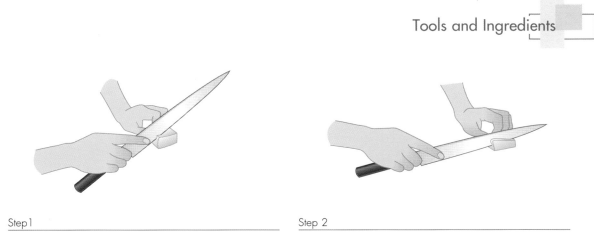

Step 1

Step 2

3. Use the knife in a sweeping action from the base to the tip (see steps 1–3).

4. Each slice will stick to the tip of the blade (see step 4).

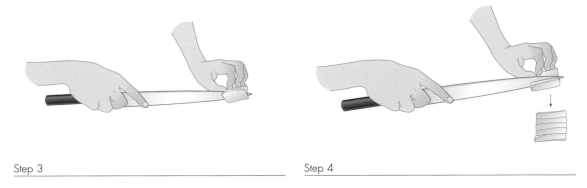

Step 3

Step 4

5. Lay the slice on its right-hand side as shown, and repeat the procedure described above.

Stocks and sauces

Basic stocks

Quality *dashi* is fundamental to Japanese cuisine. Typically, *dashi* is made of *konbu* and *hana-gatsuo*, but there is vegetarian as well as chicken *dashi*, depending on the dish it is used for. Whatever its type, *dashi* gives depth to the taste of a dish by enhancing the flavours of the ingredients. This is mainly because *dashi* itself is made of ingredients that are high in concentration of *umami*, the 'fifth taste', which is natural monosodium glutamate. *Dashi* loses its flavour quite quickly so it should be made fresh every time.

Primary dashi stock – ichiban dashi 一番だし

This is used for clear broths, the Japanese equivalent of consommé. This recipe makes 800 ml of *dashi* stock.

Preparation

- Wipe the *konbu* lightly with damp kitchen paper to remove any dust and dirt. Do not rinse with water, as the white powder on the surface is a vital source of flavour.

Measurements	Ingredients
900 ml	Cold water
10 cm square	*Konbu* (dried kelp)
30 g	*Hana-gatsuo* (dried bonito flakes)

Method

1. Place the dried *konbu* in 900 ml of cold water in an uncovered saucepan.

2. Bring slowly to the boil over a medium heat, scooping off bubbles and scum. Just before the liquid reaches boiling point, remove the *konbu* (save it for secondary *dashi* making – see the next recipe).

3. Add a ladleful of cold water to slightly cool the liquid.

4. Then add the *hana-gatsuo* (dried bonito) shavings and bring back to the boil.

5. Shut off the heat and leave the liquid undisturbed for 3–5 minutes, or until the shavings sink to the bottom of the saucepan.

6. Strain the stock through a double layer of muslin. Store in the fridge but use the same day.

Quality Points

- The stock should be clear, thin and aromatic.

Chef's Tip

- Do not throw away the used *konbu* and *hana-gatsuo*. They are useful for making a secondary *dashi* (see the following recipe).

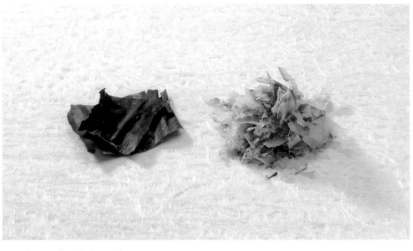

Ingredients of a *dashi* stock

Secondary dashi stock – niban dashi
二番だし

Secondary *dashi* is a general-purpose *dashi*. Here are two ways of making it.

Niban dashi recipe 1: using 'recycled' primary dashi ingredients
This recipe makes 800 ml of *dashi* stock.

Method

1. Place the water, used *konbu* and *hana-gatsuo* in a pan and bring to the boil over a medium heat. When it reaches boiling point, lower the heat to a simmer and continue to cook for 5–6 minutes.

2. Filter the stock through muslin. Store in the fridge.

Measurements	Ingredients
900 ml	Cold water
1	Used *konbu* square from the primary *dashi*
	Used *hana-gatsuo* from the primary *dashi*

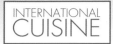

Quality Points

- The stock should be clear, thin and golden yellow, though less aromatic than the primary dashi.

Chef's Tip

- This stock is suitable for simmered dishes and miso soups.

Niban dashi recipe 2

This recipe makes 800 ml of *dashi* stock.

Preparation

- See the recipe for primary *dashi* on p. 38.

Measurements	Ingredients
900 ml	Cold water
10 cm square	*Konbu* (dried kelp)
15 g	*Hana-gatsuo* (dried bonito flakes)

Method

1. Place the water, *konbu* and *hana-gatsuo* in a pan and bring to the boil over a medium heat. When it reaches boiling point, turn down the heat to a simmer and continue to cook for 5 minutes.

2. Strain the stock through muslin. Store in the fridge.

Quality Points

- See *niban dashi* recipe 1.

Vegetarian Dashi stock 精進だし

Method

1. Rinse the dried mushrooms with water and reconstitute by soaking them in cold water for 1–2 hours, until they are soft.

2. Strain the liquid through muslin and bring to the boil. Use as required.

Measurements	Ingredients
800 ml	Water
20 g	Dried shiitake mushrooms

Quality Points

- The stock should be clear.

Chef's Tip

- It is important to use high-quality dried shiitake mushrooms. Do not soak the mushrooms for too long, otherwise the stock will end up with an overpowering flavour. Use the reconstituted mushrooms for other dishes.

Japanese chicken stock 鶏がらだし

Method

1. Pour boiling water over the chicken and rinse in cold water.

2. Chop the chicken into 2–3 cm pieces, place in a pan and cover with cold water.

3. Bring to the boil over a high heat, skim the surface, then bring down to a simmer. Continue to simmer for about 2 hours, skimming off any scum all the time, until the liquid is reduced by half. Cool and skim off the fat.

4. Strain the liquid through muslin. Use as required.

Measurements	Ingredients
150 g	Chicken bones or wings
	Boiling water (enough to thoroughly cover the chicken)
2 litres	Cold water

Quality Points

- The stock should be thin, clear and light golden in colour.

Chef's Tip

- This is a lighter chicken stock than a European equivalent. It can be combined with the general-purpose *dashi* (see p. 38) to make a richer and meatier stock.

Japanese basic vinegar dressings

All vinegar dressings work well with vegetables and seafood.

Two-flavoured vinegar (nihai-zu) dressing
二杯酢

Method

1. Combine the *dashi* and soy sauce in a pan, and bring it just to the boil.

Measurements	Ingredients
1½ tbsp	Japanese soy sauce
150 ml	*Dashi* stock or water
100 ml	Japanese rice vinegar

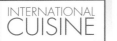

2. Mix in the vinegar and remove the pan from the heat.

3. Let the liquid cool to room temperature and then refrigerate.

Quality Points

- The dressing should be thin, vinegary and clear brown in colour.

Chef's Tip

- This is an excellent dressing for salads.

Three-flavoured vinegar (sanbai-zu) dressing
三杯酢

Method

1. Combine the *dashi*, soy sauce and caster sugar in a pan, and bring to the boil to ensure the sugar is dissolved.

2. Mix in the vinegar and remove the pan from the heat.

3. Let the liquid cool to room temperature and then refrigerate.

Measurements	Ingredients
150 ml	*Dashi* stock or water
1½ tbsp	Japanese soy sauce
1½ tbsp	Caster sugar
100 ml	Japanese rice vinegar

Quality Points

- This dressing should be vinegary, with a touch of sweetness.

Chef's Tip

- Sugar takes the sharp edge off the vinegar. This is an excellent dressing for vegetables as well as seafood salads.

Sweet vinegar (amazu) dressing 甘酢

Method

1. Combine all the ingredients in a pan and bring just to the boil, making sure the sugar is dissolved. Remove the pan from the heat.

2. Let the liquid cool to room temperature and then refrigerate.

Measurements	Ingredients
100 ml	Japanese rice vinegar
2½ tbsp	Caster sugar
Pinch	Salt
150 ml	*Dashi* stock or water

Quality Points

- The dressing should be clear, colourless and taste sweetly tart.

Chef's Tip

- This dressing goes well with a radish salad.

Dipping sauces

Ponzu sauce ポン酢

A dipping sauce for one-pot dishes such as *shabu-shabu*. *Ponzu sauce* is also suitable for seafood salads.

Method

1. Combine all the ingredients in a bowl and leave to stand for 24 hours.
2. Strain the liquid through muslin.
3. Keep refrigerated and use as required.

Quality Points

- This is a sauce with soy and citrus flavours. It should not be sour.

Measurements	Ingredients
50 ml	Freshly squeezed lemon juice
50 ml	Freshly squeezed lime juice
100 ml	Japanese soy sauce
2	*Mirin*
10 g	Bonito flakes
5 cm square	Dried *konbu*
100 ml	Japanese rice vinegar

Ground sesame sauce 胡麻だれ

This is a classic dipping sauce for *shabu-shabu*.

Method

1. In a bowl, mix the tahini with the warm *dashi*.
2. Add the remaining ingredients and mix well. Use as required.

Quality Points

- This is a smooth, nutty-flavoured sauce with the consistency of single cream.

Measurements	Ingredients
4 tbsp	Tahini
50 ml	Warm *dashi*
50 ml	Japanese rice vinegar
2½ tbsp	Japanese light soy sauce
3 tbsp	*Mirin*
Dash	Chilli oil (optional)

Chef's Tip

- Make sure the *dashi* is warm otherwise the mixture will curdle.

Miso sauce

Basic miso sauce mixture 玉味噌

Method

1. Place all the ingredients in a pan and mix well using a spatula.

2. Place the pan over a low heat and cook, stirring continuously until the mixture reaches boiling point. (Make sure it does not stick to the bottom of the pan.)

Measurements	Ingredients
200 g	White miso
1	Egg yolk
1 tbsp	Sake
1 tbsp	*Mirin*
1 tbsp	Caster sugar

3. Continue to cook for a further 2–3 minutes until the mixture resembles a thick paste.

4. Leave it to cool. Use as required.

Miso dressing 酢味噌

This sauce is excellent with blanched shellfish, legumes and seaweed salads.

Method

1. Combine the basic miso sauce mixture with the rice vinegar until the mixture is the consistency of single cream, then add the ginger juice. Taste and adjust the seasoning if necessary. Use as required.

Measurements	Ingredients
3 tbsp	Basic miso sauce mixture (see previous recipe)
1 tbsp	Japanese rice vinegar
Few drops	Ginger juice (made from squeezing freshly grated ginger)
	Salt to taste

Variation

- **Mustard-flavoured miso dressing:** Add ½ tsp of freshly prepared mustard to the above and mix well.

Soy sauce-based sauces

Sesame soy sauce ごま醤油

This sauce is often used to season blanched leaf vegetables and legumes.

Method

1. Grind the sesame seeds until they become oily.
2. Add the sugar and soy sauce, and continue to grind until they are emulsified. Use as required.

Measurements	Ingredients
3 tbsp	Toasted white sesame seeds
1½ tbsp	Caster sugar
2 tbsp	Japanese soy sauce

Mustard soy sauce 辛子醤油

This sauce goes particularly well with blanched leaf vegetables and steamed chicken or pork.

Method

1. Combine the soy sauce and *mirin*, and mix well.
2. Dissolve the mustard into the soy sauce mixture, making sure there are no lumps. Use as required.

Measurements	Ingredients
2 tbsp	Japanese soy sauce
1½ tbsp	*Mirin*
2 tsp	Freshly prepared mustard

Ginger-flavoured soy sauce 生姜醤油

This sauce is excellent for steamed chicken or fish (grilled or steamed).

Method

1. Mix the ingredients together. Use as required.

Measurements	Ingredients
2 tbsp	Japanese soy sauce
1 tsp	Ginger juice (made from squeezing freshly grated ginger)

Basic Japanese seasonings

Soy sauce, *sake*, *mirin*, rice vinegar and miso are the five key seasonings used in Japanese cuisine.

Soy sauce (醤油) – shoyu

One of the most important seasonings in Japanese cuisine, soy sauce gives flavour to the majority of Japanese dishes. For this reason, its quality is extremely important. Japanese soy sauce is naturally brewed, which gives it clarity and a hint of sweetness. There are three varieties of soy sauce – dark, light and *tamari* – and their key ingredients, aside from soy beans, are wheat, salt and *koji* (rice cultured with *aspergillus* mould). Always use Japanese soy sauce for Japanese cooking.

Dark soy sauce (濃い口醤油) – koi-kuchi shoyu

This variety is for general use. It is an essential ingredient of a variety of sauces or stocks, but is also used on its own, as in sushi. High-quality, naturally brewed soy sauce is translucent and dark brown, and has a delicate aroma. Provided it is sealed and stored in a cool place, soy sauce keeps for a long time. However, once it is opened, its flavour will be lost through oxidisation, hence it is advisable to buy it in small bottles.

Light-coloured soy sauce (薄口醤油) – usu-kuchi shoyu

Contrary to popular belief, light soy sauce has a higher sodium content than the other types, up to 2 per cent. It is typically used in dishes in which the natural flavour or original colour of the ingredients is to be maintained. In south-western-style Japanese cuisine, epitomised by *kaiseki* (see p. 6), this is the preferred soy sauce, but it is for cooking purposes only and is never used on its own.

Tamari soy sauce (たまり醤油) – tamari shoyu

This thick, dark, strong-flavoured soy sauce is usually used on its own, typically for sushi or *sashimi*. Originally a by-product of miso, this sauce is considered gluten free as it contains only the minimum amount of wheat. Select one that is dark and rich in flavour. (See dark soy sauce, above, for information on storage.)

Sake (日本酒 or 清酒) – nohon shu or sei shu

This is Japanese rice wine that is brewed from rice, *koji* (see soy sauce, above) and water. At 15 per cent proof, *sake* is brewed all over Japan where good-quality rice and spring water are available. *Sake* provides depth in flavour and taste to dishes, and is a useful tenderiser of meat or fish. It is also effective for masking a strong odour. *Sake* is primarily used for marinating, in simmered or steamed dishes and in soups. The best *sake* is reserved exclusively for drinking, but cooking *sake* should have a clean dry, non-clogging taste and a good aroma. Once the bottle as been opened, *sake* should be kept in the fridge, as its flavour and taste deteriorate rapidly. It is advisable to buy it in small quantities.

Mirin (味醂)

This is a golden-coloured, syrupy rice wine that is used exclusively for cooking. *Mirin* is an essential ingredient of grilled dishes such as *teriyaki* as it gives them their shiny gloss. *Mirin*, which is about 14 per cent proof, gives depth to a sweet taste that sugar alone cannot achieve. It is more robust than *sake*, but the alcohol is usually burnt off during cooking. Provided it is sealed and stored in a cool place, it will keep for a long time. Any white powder seen around the rim is crystallised *mirin* residue and does not affect the quality of the wine.

Japanese rice vinegar (米酢) – kome-su or yone-zu

Clear and slightly yellow in colour, Japanese rice vinegar is milder than European wine vinegar. Vinegar is frequently used in Japanese cooking – in salads and pickles – and it is an essential ingredient for marinating raw oily fish, and for sushi rice. Vinegar has an antiseptic property that helps preserve fish and rice. Seal the bottle tightly shut and store in a cool place. It will keep for a long time.

Miso (味噌)

This aromatic paste is made from crushed steamed soya beans, which are mixed together with rice, barley or bean *koji* (*aspergillous* mould) and salt, and aged for months, or up to three years. Miso that contains live enzymes is highly nutritious and has been an important source of protein for the Japanese for centuries. It is one of Japan's oldest staple foods. There are many regional varieties, each with its own distinct aroma, flavour, colour and texture.

White miso (白味噌) – shiro miso

This sweet, fine-textured 'white miso' is often used in Kyoto and south-western-style cuisine. *Saikyo* miso is the best-known example of *shiro*

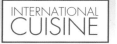

miso, and makes excellent marinades, dressings and soups. Store in an airtight container and refrigerate. It will keep for a long time, but it is advisable to buy it in small quantities as it will lose flavour.

Shinshu miso (信州味噌)

This toffee-coloured miso is the most widely used general-purpose miso. It is named after the cold mountainous region, north of Tokyo, where it originates. It is quite salty but tart. It has a variety of applications, including soups, sauces and simmered dishes (See *shiro* miso for storage advice).

Hatcho miso (八丁味噌)

This robust, chunky, chocolate-brown miso is very rich and salty. Its thickness and dark colour are characteristic of miso made with bean *koji* (*aspergillus* mould). *Hatcho* miso makes rich miso soup (p. 180). (For storage information, see *shiro* miso.)

Akadashi miso (赤だし味噌)

Chocolate brown in colour, this richly flavoured miso is a mixture of two types of miso – bean *koji* and rice *koji* – the major component being *hatcho* miso (see above). It is an essential ingredient of a topping sauce for *dengaku* dishes (see recipes on p. 109 and 113). (For storage advice, see *shiro* miso.)

Rice Products

Rice (米) – kome

Rice is the most important food in Japan. Japanese rice is the short-grain variety, but its many variants are grown throughout Japan: *koshi-hikari*, *sasa-nishiki* and *akita komachi* are the varieties best known for aroma, texture and flavour. When cooked, Japanese rice becomes slightly sticky, but fluffy on the surface and firm in texture. In Britain, most types of 'Japanese rice' available in stores are Californian grown, but are usually of very good quality. The best white rice is translucent and plump. It should be kept in a cool, airy place. In a warm climate, add a few dried whole chillies to keep insects at bay.

Glutinous rice (もち米) – mochi-gome

Short-grain glutinous rice is used primarily for making sweets and confectionery – and only occasionally in savoury dishes. The grains are opaque pearl white – not translucent. They are soaked in cold water prior to steaming. Look for plump grains and keep them in a cool, airy place.

Glutinous rice cakes (餅) – mochi

These cakes are made from steamed glutinous rice (see above). They are an essential part of Japan's New Year festive food. Steamed glutinous rice, as prepared above, is pounded to a smooth paste and then formed into small medallions or rectangular shapes. These are grilled and usually served smothered in *kinako* – toasted soya bean powder and sugar mixture (see p. 51) – or dipped in soy sauce and wrapped in *nori* seaweed. These cakes are essential ingredients of *zoni* – New Year's soup. Ready-made *mochi* are sold in packets throughout the year.

Shiratama-ko powder (白玉粉)

This is ground glutinous rice flour, used for making sweets and confectionery.

Domyoji-ko powder (道明寺粉)

This is cooked glutinous rice flour, used for making sweets and confectionery.

Joshin-ko powder (上新粉)

This is ground rice flour, used for making sweets and confectionery.

Rice bran (米糠) – kome nuka

Rice bran has many uses. It is mixed into water when boiling bamboo shoots, and also used for pickling vegetables.

Soya Bean Products

All soya bean products are extremely nutritious and have been proven to have great health benefits (as illustrated on p. 12).

Tofu (豆腐) – bean curd

Fresh tofu is made from ground soya beans. The beans are first soaked and ground, and then simmered. The resultant soy 'milk' is filtered and set by adding *nigari*, a by-product of sea salt. The custard-like curd is stored in cold water. Tofu comes in two texture types – firm cotton (*momen*) and soft silk (*kinugoshi*) – and usually comes in a 9 × 18 × 2.5cm rectangular block. Select tofu that is white, has a sheen and a faint 'cooked soya bean' smell. Purchase at retailers that keep tofu refrigerated. Any hint of sour smell indicates that it is a starting to go off.

The firm cotton type of tofu should have the texture of ricotta cheese and the silken tofu that of a loosely set custard. Cotton tofu is used for general-purpose cooking, including braising, steaming, deep-frying in

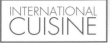

one-pot dishes; silken tofu is used primarily for broths or for eating on its own with condiments. Tofu should always be kept in water and refrigerated. Consume within a couple days of purchase. Do not freeze tofu, as it will become spongy when defrosted.

Yaki-dofu (焼き豆腐) – grilled bean curd

This lightly grilled fresh tofu has a firmer texture than cotton tofu, which makes it ideal for one-pot dishes such as *sukiyaki* (see recipe on p. 165). It is usually sold alongside fresh tofu and kept in water and refrigerated at retailers. It should be stored in the same way as fresh tofu.

Koya-dofu (高野豆腐) – dried tofu

This is traditionally dried in the open in freezing but sunny winter weather. Light yellow in colour and odourless, it comes in small rectangular pieces in packets. Closely associated with *shojin-ryori* (Buddhist vegetarian cuisine), it has an unusual spongy texture when reconstituted in warm water. Its texture and lack of taste makes *koya-dofu* ideal for simmered dishes as it quickly soaks up the seasoned liquid it is cooked in. Keep the pieces in an airtight container; they will last for a long time.

Age (揚げ) – fried bean curd

This is a deep-fried pressed tofu that looks like a thin, golden-yellow sheet. Crisp on the outside and porous inside, it is used in soups, simmered dishes or sushi. Keep refrigerated and consume within a few days of purchase.

Atsu age (厚揚げ) – thick fried bean curd

This is deep-fried fresh tofu that is thicker than *age*. It is essentially a firm tofu block with a crisp and golden exterior. It is eaten grilled with condiments or in simmered dishes. Keep refrigerated and consume within a few days of purchase.

Ganmodoki (がんもどき) – deep-fried tofu and vegetable mix

This is a deep-fried tofu and vegetable patty. Pressed tofu is crumbled, mixed with sesame seeds and shredded vegetables (carrots, mushrooms, *hijiki* seaweeds, burdock), bound with *yama-imo* (Japanese yam), made into 8 cm patties, then deep-fried. *Ganmodoki* patties have a coarse tofu texture and vegetable aroma, and are typically used in simmered or one-pot dishes. Select *ganmodoki* that does not have a strong oily smell. Keep refrigerated and consume within a few days of purchase.

Yuba (湯葉) – soya bean milk skin

This is a skin formed on the surface of soy milk during the tofu-making process. It has a very delicate texture and taste and is often associated with *shojin-royori* (Buddhist vegetarian cuisine) or *kaiseki* (see p. 6). Most *yuba* comes from Kyoto or Nikko, north of Tokyo. Although fresh *yuba* is available in Japan, it is most common in its dried form, which resembles translucent yellow paper. It comes in packets, in wide, long strips. As they are fragile, select unbroken strips, which are then softened by placing them between two wet tea towels. *Yuba* is often used in broths or simmered dishes. If placed in an airtight container, it will keep for a couple of months.

Natto (納豆) – fermented cooked soya beans

These sticky beans with their strong smell can be an acquired taste. However, *natto* is nutritious and has traditionally been served with rice and miso soup for breakfast in Kanto (the eastern region of Japan). The beans, which usually come in packets, are mixed with freshly prepared mustard, chopped spring onion and soy sauce, and spread over steamed rice. They also make an interesting filling for rolled sushi. *Natto* is usually kept in refrigerated compartments at retailers (see p. 15 for more on its health benefits).

Kinako (きな粉) – toasted soya bean powder

This soya powder with a nutty flavour is mixed with a small amount of sugar and a pinch of salt for use in sweets and confectionery. Cooked *mochi* (glutinous rice cakes) are coated with this mixture and served with green tea.

Vegetables

Arrowhead (くわい) – kuwai

An ovoid corm of a water plant, *kuwai* has a texture similar to that of a water chestnut. These corms are simmered in a seasoned stock and served as part of New Year festive food. Their brown skin is peeled and shoots removed before use. Select firm, unblemished corms.

Aubergines (茄子) – nasu

A wide variety of aubergines are used in Japanese cooking. Most Japanese aubergines are much smaller than European ones (about half the size). They have denser flesh and a sweeter flavour. They are deep-fried, sautéed, simmered, grilled, steamed or pickled in Japanese cooking. It is best to select smooth-skinned, firm, unblemished fruits.

Bamboo shoots (筍) – takenoko

Bamboo shoots, which are a sign of spring, are a popular food in Japan. Delicate in flavour and texture, the new shoots are highly sought after, which is why there are many dishes dedicated to the appreciation of new shoots and the arrival of the spring. Scrub shoots well to remove any mud and cut off the tough base. Boil the shoots in a large pan of water containing rice bran, then let them cool in the liquid. When using tinned shoots, select uncut ones and be sure to rinse them well. Remove any white residue and blanch them in hot water to remove any metallic taste before use. Keep them in fresh water and refrigerate.

Bean sprouts (もやし) – moyashi

Sprouts of mung beans, their clean and crunchy texture makes them ideal for stir-frying. They are also added to soup noodles when blanched. Sprouts should be washed first and topped and tailed before use. Select only crisp-looking ones that are white and translucent. Use on the day of purchase.

Burdock (ごぼう) – gobo

A long (50 cm), thin (2 cm in diameter at the top), muddy-looking root vegetable, burdock can be stir-fried, simmered or deep-fried as *tempura*. It has an unusual crunchy texture and a distinct earthy flavour. To prepare, scrub with a hard brush or peel off the barest minimum of the skin so as not to lose the flavour trapped just beneath the outer skin. Once cut, burdock will oxidise quickly, so immerse it in cold water. Select a thick root with dense flesh. Wrap in damp paper and store in a refrigerator.

Chinese garlic chives (韮) – nira

These are long and dark-green, grass-like leaves with a pungent aroma and fibrous texture. They are washed and cut into bite-sized pieces and often added to soup or stir-fries. Select crisp-looking, uniformly green leaves. Wrap them in damp paper to store but use them within a couple of days.

Chinese leaves (白菜) – hakusai

Barrel shaped and pale in colour, Chinese leaves are widely available throughout Britain. They have a flavour that is more delicate and sweeter than that of European cabbage and are ideal for stir-fried, simmered or one-pot dishes. Select heavy ones with tight heads. They keep well if wrapped in damp paper and stored in a cool place.

Cucumber (胡瓜) – kyuri

Japanese cucumbers are smaller, thinner skinned and have a sweeter flavour than European varieties; they also have fewer seeds. Lebanese cucumbers, available at British stores, are the nearest to the Japanese variety. They are essential ingredients of sushi, Japanese salads and pickles.

When using ordinary cucumbers, scoop out the seeds completely and remove the skin.

Daikon radish (大根)

This root vegetable, which looks like a large white carrot, is known as mooli in Britain. A type of radish, it is used extensively in Japanese cookery. It is normally about 30 cm in length and 10 cm in diameter, but comes in many varieties and sizes in Japan. Although it is available throughout the year, it tastes best in winter. It is peeled and grated raw, and used as a condiment; or it may be cut up and simmered in a stock. Small ones are pickled whole. Select a firm, heavy and unblemished root. When it is cut horizontally, the surface should be moist, smooth and fine textured. (Holes at the centre indicate that it has dried out and is no longer suitable for consumption.) Wrap in damp paper and store in a cool place. It will keep for a few days.

Edible chrysanthemum leaves (春菊) – shungiku

These leaves are deeply lobed and brighter green than the garden variety. Their slightly bitter taste makes them suitable for one-pot dishes and soups when used in small quantities. Select crisp, undamaged leaves, and remove the central stalks. Keep them wrapped in damp paper and consume within a couple of days of purchase.

Enokidake (えのきだけ) mushrooms

These are about 10 cm in length, creamy off-white in colour with uniform thin stems with tiny caps. Unlike European mushrooms, these are tree mushrooms and have a fruity smell and sweeter taste. They are used to add texture and a hint of sweet flavour to soups, stir-fries and one-pot dishes. They need to be cooked for only a couple of minutes otherwise they will lose their flavour and shape. Select firm, unblemished ones with caps and stems intact. Once the packet is opened, use the contents the same day.

Ginger (生姜) – shoga

Ginger is always used fresh in Japanese cooking, never in its powdered or preserved form. The ginger rhizome is washed, skinned and grated, and used together with its juice as flavouring. The peel is useful in simmered dishes. Ginger is shredded when used as a garnish and sliced for making pickles. Select young, plump and smooth, thin-skinned rhizomes; old ones have a dark and shrivelled skin. Keep them wrapped and stored in the vegetable compartment of a fridge.

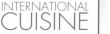

Gingko nuts (銀杏) – ginnan

These are the nuts of the female gingko tree. Encased in hard, white shells around 1.5 cm in diameter, these nuts are yellow-green and have a strong flavour and chewy texture. They are often added to *chawan-mushi* (a savoury custard cup) or grilled on a skewer, *yakitori* style. The outer shells are cracked open, and the nuts inside are boiled; their transparent skin is then removed before use. Select those with unbroken shells. They will keep for weeks in a refrigerator.

Green soya beans (枝豆) – edamame

These are young soya beans in pods. They are boiled, sprinkled with salt and served as a snack or side dish. Fresh ones usually come in packets, or attached to stems, but in Britain they are usually only available frozen. Select firm, full pods. Fresh ones should be wrapped in newspaper and stored in the vegetable compartment of a fridge.

Japanese yam (山芋) – Yama-imo and naga-imo

The nearest equivalent to these tubers are yams. Beige and hairy-skinned, they are long and wooden stick-like, or flat and hand-shaped, and are used extensively in Japanese cookery. When they are peeled and grated, they will develop an unusually viscous texture. They are eaten raw in this way or used as a binding agent in *ganmodoki* (see tofu products, p. 50) in order to give it fluffiness. At the greengrocers they are stored in sawdust to stop them drying out.

Kabocha (南瓜) squash

This is a round and flat squash, about 20 cm in diameter, with dark-green skin. The flesh is deep yellow and has a fine texture. This vegetable is widely available in Britain. It is cut into small segments and the seeds removed, and is either simmered or deep-fried. Cooked *kabocha* has a sweet and chestnut-like flavour and texture. Select heavy squashes with unblemished skin. Keep in a cool place and use within a week.

Komatsuna (小松菜)

This is another leafy vegetable, indigenous to Japan. It is about 20 cm in height with long green leaves and thick stalks. It is grown as mustard spinach in Britain, though it is unrelated to spinach and more akin to radish. It has a refreshing and subtle flavour, and is eaten stir-fried, blanched or dressed in soy sauce. Select crisp-looking leaves with firm stalks. Use on day of purchase.

Lotus root (蓮根) – renkon

This is the root of a water plant that is muddy beige and tubular shaped with hollow channels running through its entire length. Each root is about 7 cm in diameter and 20 cm in length, but it is often sold in segments. It is prized for its crunchy texture and is stir-fried, simmered, pickled in vinegar or deep-fried as *tempura*. To prepare, wash thoroughly to remove any mud. Peel the skin, making sure to immerse the root in water to prevent discolouration. It is usually used sliced. It will become whiter if it is immersed in a water and vinegar mixture. Select firm roots without any blemishes, which indicate decay. Keep them wrapped in paper and store in a cool place.

Matsutake (松茸) mushrooms

One might say *matsutake* are to the Japanese what truffles are to Europeans. They are available only for a few weeks in the autumn. As they grow only in the wild and in red pine woods, they have a wonderful pine flavour and a unique meaty texture. For these reasons they are extremely expensive. These mushrooms are most sought-after before the caps open so that the pine flavour is concentrated within. They are dark brown, 10–15 cm in height and have very thick stems and dense caps. There are a number of soups and dishes that have been devised especially for these premier mushrooms. Caps as well as the stems are sliced and eaten in broths, grilled *en papillote*, or in a special rice dish.

Mizuna (水菜)

This vegetable is widely available as salad leaves in Britain. They are eaten blanched in Japan in the same way as spinach or *komatsuna*. Select crisp-looking leaves. Use on the day of purchase.

Myoga (茗荷)

Shoots and flower buds of this Japanese woodland plant are shredded for use in salads or garnishes. The aromatic and crunchy shoots add a touch of spring to dishes. They are imported to Britain but may not be readily available at retailers. If you find them, select ones that are firm and crisp looking. Keep them refrigerated and wrapped in damp paper, and use within a few days of purchase.

Nameko (なめこ) mushrooms

These are about 5 cm in length with amber-coloured small caps, which have a gelatinous coating. They are also tree mushrooms. Although they are usually sold in jars or airtight packets in Japan, they are available fresh in Britain. They have a woody flavour and are most commonly used in miso soup or a salad with grated *daikon* radish (mooli). Select firm ones with even-sized caps and the mycelium attached. They require only a few minutes of cooking, otherwise their delicate flavour is lost. Use on the day of purchase.

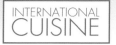

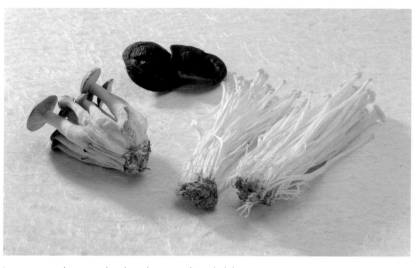

Japanese mushrooms: shiitake, *shimeji* and *enokidakei*

Sato-imo (里芋)

Known as eddoe in Britain, these are small, brown, hairy-skinned and ovoid tubers. A variety of *taro*, they are important ingredients of a number of simmered dishes. Peel the hairy skin thickly and soak them in water to prevent them discolouring. Once peeled, *sato-imo* tubers get slimy, and may make your hands itchy. However, they have a subtly sweet taste and a rich, velvety texture when cooked. Select firm ones without any wormholes. Keep wrapped in paper and store in a cool place. Use within two to three days.

Shiitake (椎茸) mushrooms

The most widely used mushrooms in Japanese cookery, these are sold fresh or dried. Shiitake are so called because they grow on the shii tree, a type of Japanese oak. The dried type should be soaked in water and reconstituted before use. The soaking liquid can be added to a stock for flavour. The shiitake's meaty flavour and texture makes it suitable for any type of cooking – including broths, stir-fries, deep-fries, and simmered, steamed or one-pot dishes, or certain kinds of sushi. Fresh shiitake mushrooms should be dark brown with no blemishes on the cap or underside, and should have a good mushroom aroma. The best dried shiitake mushrooms have thick, black, wrinkled caps. Fresh ones will keep a few days in moist conditions. The dried type will keep for a few months if kept in an airtight container. (See p. 16 for information on the health benefits of shiitake mushrooms.)

Shimeji (しめじ) mushrooms

These have grey caps and are similar in size to *nameko*. They have a subtle, delicious flavour, and are used for soups, stir-fries or rice dishes.

As with other mushrooms, they need only be cooked for a few minutes. Select firm ones that have even-sized caps with the mycelium attached, and that have a good mushroom aroma.

Small Japanese green peppers (獅子唐辛子) — shishi-togarashi

These are small (5–7 cm in height) green peppers that look like green chillies. They are sweet but slightly hot. These peppers are grilled whole and used as a garnish or served with *yakitori*. Select firm, unblemished ones. Keep them refrigerated and use within three to four days.

Spinach (ほうれん草) — horen-so

Japanese spinach, unlike the European variety, has bigger and thicker leaves, which come attached to their long stalks. The Italian variety is closest to the Japanese type. The leaves, as well as the stalks, are always blanched first and served with a soy or sesame-based sauce. Select crisp-looking leaves with firm stalks.

Spring onions (葱) — negi

Traditional Japanese onions are longer (40 cm), thicker and sweeter than the spring onions available in Britain. Used extensively in cookery, they are chopped finely and served as a condiment with one-pot dishes, or sliced thinly and blanched for garnishing. They are also added to soups, or stir-fried or simmered with other foods. Select firm, crispy-looking bunches with roots attached and free of discoloured outer skins. Wrap in damp paper and refrigerate. They will keep for three or four days.

Stem ginger (新生姜) — shin-shoga

This is a young ginger rhizome and its shoot. Pale yellow in colour, the rhizome has a clear, thin skin and a long, pink, stemmed shoot. It is usually pickled in vinegar and used as a garnish.

Sweet potatoes (薩摩芋) — satsuma-imo

This tuber is a popular ingredient in Japanese cookery. There are many different varieties but Japanese sweet potatoes have purple skin, dense yellow flesh and a sweeter, more chestnut-like taste than other varieties. The Jamaican sweet potatoes that are sold in Britain are the nearest to the Japanese variety. They are simmered, deep-fried or stone-baked. Scrub clean before use and soak in water to prevent discoloration. Select unblemished, heavy potatoes. Use within a few days of purchase.

Takuwan (沢庵)

This is a pickled white radish. It is salted, sun-dried and then pickled in rice bran. Its yellow colour comes from turmeric, which is used for the colouring. It is often used as a filling for sushi rolls and is usually sold in a vacuum pack. Once the package is opened, keep refrigerated and consume within a couple of days.

Turnips (蕪) – kabu

Japanese turnips are pure white with a smooth, thin skin. About 10 cm in diameter, they look like a white radish but are sweeter, moister and smoother textured. Often they are sliced thinly for use in salads or pickles, but there are also sophisticated simmered dishes using these turnips. They are usually sold with their long leaves attached, which can be eaten stir-fried.

Wood ear mushrooms (木耳) – kikurage

Resembling the dry black bark of a tree, these mushrooms are rarely available fresh. They are soaked in tepid water until soft and translucent before use. *Kikurage* in Japanese means 'tree jelly fish' and this is precisely what the texture is like – crisp but floppy. The mushrooms are prized for this unique texture and are often added to simmered dishes and stir-fries. Select the ones that are even in size and black in colour. If placed in an airtight container, they will keep for a long time.

Herbs

Kinome (木の芽) leaves – young leaves of the prickly ash

Kinome leaves are the new leaves of the deciduous Japanese prickly ash tree. These young leaves, which are available only in the spring, are used widely in Japanese cuisine at that time of the year for seasonal effects. Being highly fragrant, they are used in broths, or in simmered, grilled and tofu dishes to add a hint of citrus bouquet. The *kinome* (prickly ash) plant grows in the British climate, but it is difficult to obtain the leaves at British stores. If you can get them, wrap them in damp cotton wool and store them in the fridge. They will keep for a few days.

Mitsuba (三つ葉) – trefoil

A member of the parsley family, trefoil has long (about 30 cm), pale-green stalks with light-green leaves attached to each in threes; hence the Japanese name 'three leaves', or *mitsuba*. It has a delicate aromatic flavour, and is used in broths, Japanese salads, and steamed or one-pot dishes, both as a flavouring and a garnish. Since it is only used fresh, it is usually sold with the roots attached in Japan in order to maintain its freshness. Select a bunch with strong, firm stems and young leaves. Wrap in damp paper and keep refrigerated. It will keep for about a week. Do not substitute with coriander, which, although similar in appearance, has an entirely different, overpowering aroma.

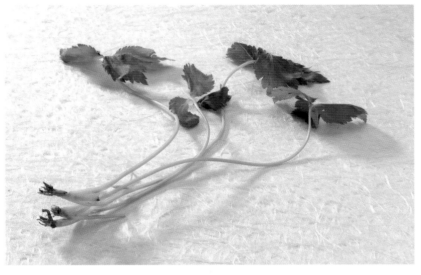

Mitsuba leaves

Shiso (紫蘇) leaves – perilla

Shiso, a member of the mint family, is a highly aromatic herb. Its leaves, which look similar to those of the nettle, are used as garnishes or a condiment. *Shiso* is grown in Britain and comes in two types – green and purple – the former being more common than the latter. The purple leaves, which resemble purple basil, are used primarily for making pickled plums (see *ume-boshi*, p. 67). These leaves give a beautiful magenta colour with a hint of aniseed flavour to them. Select fresh-looking leaves. Wrap them in damp paper and keep them refrigerated. Use within a week of purchase.

Dry Ingredients

Adzuki beans (小豆)

This is a dark-red coloured small pulse, which is used mainly for sweet red bean paste for Japanese confectionery. It is also added when making festive red steamed rice. It is highly nutritious (see p. 17). Soak the beans overnight before cooking. Select plump, unbroken beans. Store them in an airy, cool, dry place.

Fu (麩) – wheat gluten

Fu is wheat gluten made from strong wheat flour, typically used in soups, soup noodles and one-pot dishes. High in protein and low in starch, *fu* 'cakes' in a variety of shapes, some decorative, are usually available in dried form. The wheat gluten is softened in tepid water for up to ten minutes and excess liquid is pressed out before use. The cakes are sold in

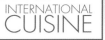

packets. Select firm, unbroken ones. If stored in an airtight container, they will keep for a long time.

Hana-gatsuo (花鰹)

These are ready-made shavings of *katsuo-bushi* (see p. 61), and are essential ingredients of *dashi* stock. The translucent, salmon-pink shavings usually come in large packets. Select fresh-looking, pale-pink ones. Keep them dry in an airtight container, as their flavour and aroma will disappear rapidly once the packet is opened.

Hijiki (ひじき) seaweeds

These are dark-brown, dried twig-like seaweeds that have a slightly chewy texture. Typically, *hijiki* seaweeds are simmered in a seasoned stock with root vegetables and tofu products such as *age* (fried bean curd). When soaked in water to reconstitute, they expand by nearly eight times. They are sold in packets. Select dark seaweeds with a slight sheen. Keep them dry in an airtight container. They will keep for a long time.

Ito-kezuri (糸削り)

These are the finer, thread-like shavings of *katsuo-bushi* (see below) sold in packets. They are used primarily for garnishing vegetable dishes but add a refined texture and subtle flavour to almost any dish. Select fine, pale-pink shavings. Keep them dry in an airtight container so as not to lose their flavour. Finger-crushed *hana-gatsuo* (see above) is a practical substitute for these expensive shavings.

Kanpyo (干瓢) – dried gourd shavings

These dry, white, long ribbons are the shavings of the Japanese *yugao* gourd. Before they are reconstituted in tepid water, they are washed in cold water and rubbed with salt. They expand nearly ten times in volume when reconstituted. The ribbons are boiled, then simmered in a seasoned stock for use as a sushi filling. They are sold in packets. Select firm, clean-looking ribbons. Keep them dry in an airtight container. They will keep for a long time.

Kanten (寒天) – agar-agar

Made from a red seaweed called *tengusa*, *kanten* is the traditional setting agent for Japanese sweets and confectionery. Its 42°C setting point and 82°C melting point are much higher than those of gelatine, but it gives a firmer texture and delicate flavour. *Kanten* comes in porous translucent sticks, thin strips or powder. The dry sticks and strips are first soaked in water to let them expand. After the water has been squeezed out, *kanten* pieces are then placed in clean cold water in a saucepan and simmered until they dissolve. Select fresh-looking, unbroken sticks or strips. Keep them dry in an airtight container so that they last a long time without discolouring.

Katsuo-bushi (鰹節) – dried bonito fillets

The dried fillet of the bonito fish is one of the indispensable ingredients of *dashi* stock. Bonito fillets are dried for a long time by traditional means until they resemble pieces of hard wood. They are planed and the shavings become the basis of *dashi* stock. Fresh shavings have a wonderful smoky aroma, but ready-shaved *hana-gatsuo* (see above), sold in packets, is most widely used. *Katsuo-bushi*, the original wood-like block, will keep indefinitely if kept in a dry place, but *hana-gatsuo* won't. There are two types of *katsuo-bushi*: white fillet (back) and dark (belly). The white fillet is more expensive.

Kezuri-bushi (削り節)

Another name for *hana-gatsuo* (see above).

Konbu (昆布) – kelp seaweed

Konbu, which has a high concentration of natural monosodium glutamate, is one of the essential ingredients of *dashi* stock. Kelp plants grow to over 5 m in height in the cold sea of the northern Japanese region of Hokkaido, where they are harvested, dried and packaged. They are deep olive-green in colour and, in the packet, look like stiff dried sheets. Never wash or rinse them – just wipe with a damp cloth if necessary, as the white powder on the surface is a source of flavour and not dust. When making *dashi*, a piece of *konbu* is put in a pan full of cold water and placed on the stove. There are several quality grades in *konbu*. Select thick sheets that are dark olive green. Keep them dry in an airtight container or freeze in a plastic bag. They will keep for a couple of months. (See p. 16 for information on the health benefits of kelp.)

Nori (海苔) seaweed

Nori is dried marine algae made into the standard 20.5 × 17.5 cm sheets. Deep dark green in colour, its crisp texture and sea aroma complement rice extremely well. *Nori* is what rolled sushi is wrapped in, as are rice balls and *mochi* rice cakes (see p. 49). *Nori* sheets can be toasted immediately before use but they are commonly available ready toasted. Look for deep dark-green sheets that are dense in texture. Once they lose crispness, all the flavour and the taste disappear. If placed in an airtight container, they will keep for a couple of months. (See p. 16 for information on the health benefits of *nori*.)

Panko (パン粉) breadcrumbs

These breadcrumbs, made of bleached wheat flour, dextrose and vegetable oil, are essential for *tonkatsu*. Flakier and lighter than ordinary crumbs, they brown better and do not get soggy – ideal for making crisp, golden-brown deep-fried dishes. These Japanese-style crumbs are sold in packets. Select packets containing pale and uniform crumbs. If kept in an airtight container, they will last a long time.

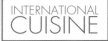

Wakame (若布) seaweed

When dried, *wakame* resembles small, dark-green, shrivelled-up leaves. (In Japan, salted fresh *wakame* is available at fishmongers.) Soft but crunchy in texture, *wakame* is a popular ingredient of miso soup or Japanese salads. When reconstituted in water, it expands by nearly eight times. Cut away the hard central stalks before use. Select thick-leaved *wakame* that is dark green in colour. It comes in packets. Keep it dry in an airtight container. It should last for a few months. (See p. 16 for information on the health benefits of *wakame*.)

Traditional Japanese Noodles

Noodles are an extremely popular food in Japan, a country with more than 300 years of noodle-eating tradition. Quick, inexpensive and readily available, a bowl or plate of noodles remains a popular lunch or a light evening meal throughout Japan to this day. In fact, along with *nigiri-zushi*, noodles are the traditional fast food of Japan.

Japanese noodles are made of either wheat flour – as in *udon*, *kishimen*, *hiyamugi* or *somen* – or buckwheat flour – as in *soba*. Wheat noodles are particularly popular in the south-west of Japan, and buckwheat noodles are eaten in Tokyo and the north-east. This is probably because the buckwheat plant grows in the relatively colder climate of the north. In the south-west, meanwhile, there is a strong tradition of wheat noodles, which has given rise to at least four distinct types of wheat flour noodle, as mentioned above. *Udon* and *soba* are available fresh or dry, whereas all other types of wheat noodle are available only dry. All noodles are delicious either eaten cold with dipping sauce and condiments or, in the case of soup noodles, with toppings. Dried Japanese noodles keep for a long time in the packet or if stored in an airtight container.

Wheat noodles
Udon (うどん)

These are round or flat white noodles made of wheat flour, salt and water. They are available either fresh or dry. *Udon* noodles come in a range of thicknesses and lengths, and are eaten cold, dipped in sauce, usually with the condiments of grated fresh ginger and finely chopped spring onions. Sanuki (Kagawa prefecture in south-west Japan) and Inaniwa (north-west Japan) are best known for their top-quality *udon*.

Inaniwa udon (稲庭うどん)

These ultra-fine handmade noodles, produced exclusively in Akita prefecture, northern Japan, may well be the most expensive noodles in the world. Originally developed in the seventeenth century for the local warlord, these noodles were available only to the Imperial Household

Agency until the end of the Second World War. To this day, these noodles are made entirely by hand, using traditional methods which give them their unique texture. *Inaniwa udon* is on the menu of exclusive restaurants in Japan and elsewhere, where they are often served cold with dipping sauce and condiments. These noodles are only available dry.

Kishimen (きしめん)

These are the wide, ribbon-like variation of *udon* developed in Nagoya, east of Kyoto. They are cooked and served the same way as *udon*, but are only available dry.

Somen (素麺)

These are very fine and delicate white noodles made from hard-wheat dough containing sesame or other types of vegetable oil. They are popular summer noodles, eaten cold, dipped in sauce with grated ginger as a condiment. But they are also eaten hot in a clear soup, in the same way as *udon* in south-west Japan. Miwa (Nara prefecture), Ibo (Himeji prefecture) and Shodoshima Island (Shikoku region) – all in south-west Japan – are best known for their top-quality *somen*. *Tamago somen* (egg *somen*) is a variation that contains egg yolk. Warm yellow in colour, these noodles are used primarily as a garnish in clear soup.

Hiyamugi (冷麦)

They are almost identical to *somen* (see above) but are slightly thicker and do not contain vegetable oil. Their texture, as a result, is slightly softer.

Buckwheat noodles

Soba (蕎麦)

Flour made from buckwheat grains, which are dark brown and triangular shaped, is the primary ingredient of *soba*. However, wheat is usually added to give the elasticity required for making noodles. The dark-brown *soba* that contains buckwheat bran is called *inaka soba* (country-style noodle) and the more popular light-brown one is called *sarashina soba*. Some of the fresh *soba* requires less than a minute of boiling time, but even the more common dry types usually take only a few minutes to cook. *Soba* comes in a variety of thicknesses, as does *udon*.

Cha soba (茶蕎麦) – tea soba

Matcha (powdered green tea) is added to make green *cha soba*, for the flavour. This may be eaten cold in the same way as *soba*, or used as a garnish in clear soup.

Condiments

Dai-dai (ダイダイ) – dai-dai citron

The juice of this orange-sized and coloured citrus fruit is not as sharp as that of *yuzu*, but they both have similar applications. *Dai-dai* juice makes excellent *ponzu* sauce (see recipe on p. 43) and other Japanese vinegar dressings. Unlike *sudachi* or *yuzu*, its rind is rarely used.

Mustard (辛子) – karashi

This Japanese mustard is very similar to English mustard but slightly hotter. It is always freshly made from powder. It is a condiment and flavouring for sauces. It is prepared in the same way as powdered *wasabi* (see below). For the recipes in this book, substitute with English mustard powder.

Sansho (山椒) – sansho powder

This pungent greenish-beige powder is not pepper but it can be quite hot. It tastes tangy with a citrus undertone. Made from the ground pods of the Japanese prickly ash, *sansho* powder is often sprinkled over grilled eels or *yakitori* to counterbalance their oiliness. The leaves, known as *kinome*, are used as garnishes (see herbs, p. 58). *Sansho* powder comes in a small screw-topped bottle. It is advisable to buy it in small quantities as it loses flavour through oxidisation.

Sesame seeds (胡麻) – goma

Both black and white sesame seeds are used frequently in Japanese cooking. They are dry-toasted to bring out the nutty and aromatic flavours before use. Black seeds have a stronger flavour than white ones. They are used whole as garnishes and coarsely ground for sauces. Whole seeds are often mixed with toasted salt for use in rice dishes. Select clean, unbroken seeds that are not oily in appearance. Store them in an airtight container and they will keep for a long time.

Shichimi togarashi (七味唐辛子) – seven-spice pepper

As the English translation suggests, this colourful condiment is a collection of seven dried and coarsely ground spices – red chilli flakes, ground *sansho* pods, hemp seeds, dried mandarin orange peel, white poppy seeds, *nori* seaweed and black sesame seeds. It is sprinkled over soup noodles (*udon* or *soba*) or *yakitori* at the table to add piquancy. It comes in a small screw-topped bottle. It is advisable to buy it in small quantities, as oxidisation causes the flavour to deteriorate.

Sudachi (スダチ) – sudachi citron

This tiny, lime-green citrus fruit, grown in south-west Japan, is highly sought after for its sharp but aromatic juice and rind. It is squeezed over grilled dishes to add a tangy flavour, and the rind is grated and mixed into vinegar dressings.

Wasabi (わさび)

Wasabi is unique to Japan, and contrary to popular belief it is not related to the European horseradish. The plant grows in cold and clear streams, and its gnarled root is peeled and grated with an ultra-fine grater to accompany *sashimi* and *nigiri-zushi*. It is pale green in colour. As fresh wasabi roots are expensive and in short supply, the powder is widely used and ready-made paste is also available in a tube. To prepare powdered *wasabi*, add a small amount of cold water to make a stiff smooth paste, cover and allow to stand for five minutes to develop the pungent flavour. Powdered *wasabi* will keep in a tin for a long time.

Yuzu (柚子) – yuzu citron

This is a uniquely Japanese citrus fruit that is yellow in colour and about the size of a mandarin orange. The presence of *yuzu* is a sign of winter in the Japanese culinary calendar. Its unique, pungent aroma is concentrated in the rind. The rind makes an effective garnish or gives unique flavour to soup. It is also added to *soba* soups, salads, miso sauces and simmered dishes. The freshly squeezed juice is mixed with vinegar when making salad dressings. Freeze-dried *yuzu* rind is available. Although weaker in aroma, the dried version is a useful substitute.

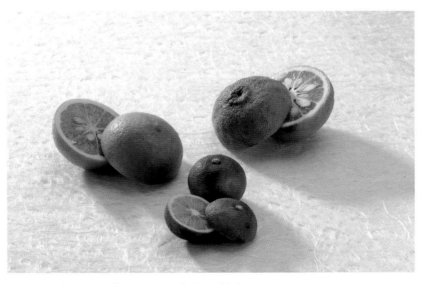

Japanese culinary citrus fruits: *yuzu*, *sudachi* and *kabosu*

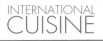

Oils and flours

Oil (油) – abura

Rapeseed, corn and safflower oil are most commonly used for stir-frying and deep-frying in Japan. They are preferred over other oils because they do not have a strong flavour and therefore do not interfere with the main ingredients. They also give a lighter finish to fried dishes. Sunflower or any other light vegetable oil is equally suitable. Keep a bottle sealed and stored in a cool place in order to minimise oxidisation.

Sesame oil (胡麻油) – goma abura

This is a seasoning oil that gives a nutty flavour to dishes. It should be sprinkled over them just before serving. Select the clear, lighter-brown oil that is extracted from lightly toasted sesame seeds. Keep the bottle sealed and store it in a cool place. However, as flavour will be lost through oxidisation, it is advisable to buy only a small bottle at time.

Potato starch (片栗粉) – katakuri-ko

This is the most common thickener in Japanese cooking, and it is also used as dusting flour for deep-frying. Sold in packets, the starch should be kept in an airtight container.

Kuzu (葛)

This flour, extracted from *kuzu* root, is the traditional thickener used in Japanese cooking. It is also used in making confectionery. This fine and expensive flour gives a velvety consistency and shiny gloss to sauces and clear soups. As a result, it is preferred over other thickening agents for refined cuisine. However, being very fine, it can get lumpy if not handled with care. The flour is sold in packets. If placed in an airtight container, it will keep for a long time.

Other Products

Beni-shoga (紅生姜)

This is red-coloured salted ginger, and comes either sliced or shredded in a packet or a jar. It is used as a garnish or a filling for rice dishes. Most *beni-shoga* is artificially coloured, but natural, red plum-coloured varieties are also available. If kept in a jar, it will last for a few months.

Ito-konnyaku (糸こんにゃく)

Another name for thread *konnyaku* (see *shira-taki* and *konnyaku*, below).

Kamaboko (蒲鉾)

This is a generic name for Japanese fish cake made from puréed white fish, starch and seasonings. *Kamaboko* comes in a variety of shapes and sizes, but the most popular kind – *ita-kamaboko* – which is served mounted on a small rectangular piece of wood, requires no more preparation than slicing. Sliced *kamaboko* is eaten with *wasabi* and soy sauce, and is an essential part of the Japanese New Year's meal. Sliced *kamaboko* is often added to clear soups or steamed dishes to add flavour, garnish and texture. *Ita-kamaboko* is sold wrapped in thick plastic paper and is kept refrigerated at retailers. Select a firm piece. Keep it refrigerated at all times and eat within a couple of days of purchase.

Konnyaku (こんにゃく) – devil's tongue jelly

This is a gelatinous, grey rectangular (15 × 8 × 4 cm) cake. It is made from the starchy root of devil's tongue. The roots are cooked, pounded and mixed with milk of lime to coagulate, and then formed into cakes or threads. *Konnyaku* is boiled first to remove its inherent smell, then pounded to make the texture porous so that it will easily absorb the flavours of the foods it is simmered with. *Konnyaku* has little flavour or taste, but its firm jelly-like texture adds a new dimension to simmered or one-pot dishes. It is also available in thread-like forms of *shira-taki* or *ito-konnyaku*. Fresh *konnyaku* is sold in a water packet, and can be found in a retailer's refrigerated section. After purchase, keep refrigerated and use within a week. (See p. 15 for information on the health benefits of *konnyaku*.)

Shira-taki (しらたき) – thread konnyaku

This is a threaded version of *konnyaku* (see above). It is an essential ingredient of *sukiyaki* (see p. 165 for recipe) and is widely used in simmered dishes.

Umeboshi (梅干) – pickled red plums

These are green plums pickled in salt and purple *shiso* (perilla) leaves. They are among the most popular pickles in Japan, often eaten with steamed white rice and *nori* seaweed, but they also make an interesting seasoning in simmered dishes. These plums, which are closely related to apricots, are harvested in June. After preliminary pickling in salt, they are sun-dried, rubbed in *shiso* leaves, which gives them their magenta colour, and pickled for a further six months, or up to a year. Select plump and succulent-looking ones. They will keep a long time if stored in a container in a cool place.

Recipes

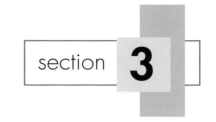

section **3**

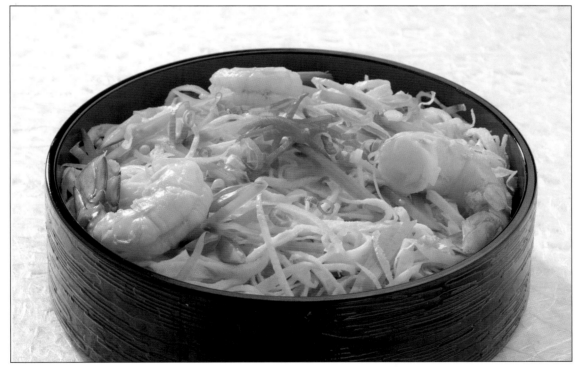

Scattered sushi, Osaka style (see p. 72)

chapter 9

GETTING STARTED: BEGINNERS' RECIPES

All recipes serve four unless stated otherwise.

Dedicated to beginners, this chapter focuses on traditional dishes that are relatively simple to make, and for which the ingredients and equipment required are available in Europe. The dishes are arranged into lunch and dinner menus, as follows, for practical purposes.

Sushi lunch

Chirashi-zushi (scattered sushi) Osaka style

Beaten egg soup

Chicken teriyaki *dinner*

Teriyaki chicken

Stir-fried bean sprouts, shiitake mushrooms and spring onions

Cucumber and *wakame* seaweed with Japanese vinegar dressing

Chicken broth

Steamed rice

Fish dinner

Grilled marinated salmon with grated *daikon* radish

Kimpira carrots

Blanched okra with Japanese vinegar dressing

Tofu and *wakame* miso soup

Mushroom rice

Tofu dinner

Tofu steak with Japanese mushroom and ginger sauce

Stir-fried boiled quails' eggs, sugar-snap peas and spring onions

Asparagus with chilli-flavoured sesame dressing

Potato and onion miso soup

Jade rice

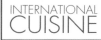
Sushi lunch

Chirashi-Zushi (Scattered Sushi) Osaka Style
大阪風ちらし寿し

To make the basic mixed sushi rice

1. Place the cool sushi rice in a large mixing bowl.

2. Sprinkle the toasted sesame seeds over the rice and mix well, taking care not to crush the grains.

3. Add the lemon peel, followed by the ginger and the white sesame seeds, and mix well. Make sure the two types of sesame seed, lemon peel and ginger are evenly mixed into the rice.

To make the topping and garnishes

1. Flake the smoked trout with a fork and put aside.

2. Shell, de-vein and wash the prawns. Poach them in slightly salted water until they just turn pink and plunge them into iced water to arrest cooking. Dry them and put them aside.

3. Mix the eggs with the sugar and a pinch of salt. Strain the egg mixture so it will make smooth omelettes. Heat an 18–20 cm skillet over a medium heat. Grease the pan very lightly with an oil-soaked kitchen towel. Test the pan for temperature by dropping a bit of egg in the centre. It should sizzle. Pour just enough mixture into the pan to make a paper-thin omelette. Turn down the heat, and when the surface of the egg mixture is almost dry, quickly flip it over. Cook for another 4–5 seconds until the surface is dry. Remove it from the pan and leave it on a plate to cool.

Measurements	Ingredients
2 cups (400 ml)	Sushi rice (see p. 91 for recipe)
Basic rice mix	
2 tbsp	Toasted black sesame seeds
2 thin strips	Lemon peel without pith, cut into 2 mm julienne strips
2 tbsp	Sushi ginger, chopped to the same size as the cooked grains of rice
2 tbsp	White sesame seeds
Topping	
2 fillets	Smoked trout, skinned and boned
4 medium-sized	Prawns
2	Eggs
1 tsp	Caster sugar
Pinch	Salt
6	Mangetout, blanched, cut into diagonal 2 mm strips
3	Spring onions, very thinly sliced
Garnish	
5 cm	*Nori* seaweed sheet, cut into 1 mm strips

4. Re-grease the pan and use the remaining egg mixture to make more omelettes. Do not stack them up while they are hot, as they will stick together. For the 'golden string' garnish, stack up these omelettes once they have cooled down and cut them crosswise into very thin strings (1–2 mm in width).

To assemble and serve

Sprinkle the flaked trout, spring onions (the white part only) and mangetout strips over the mixed rice. Then cover thickly with the omelette strings. Scatter prawns and spring onions (the green part) over the top and garnish with *nori* seaweed.

Beaten Egg Soup かき玉汁

This is a very popular soup in Japan and goes well with most dishes. Traditionally, this soup is made solely with *dashi* stock but in the following recipe this has been combined with chicken stock.

Method

1. Mix the *dashi* and chicken stock in a pan and bring to the boil over a medium heat, then reduce the heat to a simmer.

2. Add the salt and soy sauce to the stock.

3. While the stock is simmering, stir in the *sake* and the dissolved potato starch.

4. Stir until it thickens. Then continue to cook until just before boiling point.

5. Take the soup off the heat and slowly pour in the beaten egg in a thin stream, forming a coil over the surface of the soup as you do so. Let the egg start to set for 30 seconds to 1 minute. Stir the soup gently with a fork to separate the egg into threads.

6. Add the ginger to the soup and mix well.

7. Serve the soup hot in individual bowls, garnishing each one with a pinch of the spring onion strips.

Measurements	Ingredients
400 ml	*Dashi* stock
400 ml	Chicken stock
1 tsp	Salt
⅔ tsp	Japanese light soy sauce
1 tsp	*Sake*
1 tsp	Potato starch dissolved with 1 tbsp of water
1	Egg, beaten
¼ tsp	Ginger, freshly grated
Garnish	
1	Spring onion, cut into pieces 1 mm wide, 2.5 cm long

Quality Points

- The soup should be smooth and have the consistency of single cream.

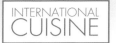

Japan

Chicken teriyaki dinner

Teriyaki, meaning 'a shiny grilled dish', is usually a grilled or pan-fried fish or chicken glazed with a sauce made of soy sauce, sugar, *mirin* and *sake*. Oily fish, such as yellowtail, or chicken works well with this method of cooking as its oil gives an impressive 'shine'. Authentic *teriyaki*, which has a subtle and delicate flavour, bears little resemblance to the '*teriyaki*' beef that is often served at restaurants in the West.

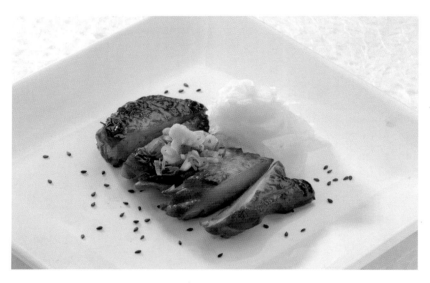

Teriyaki Chicken
鶏肉の照り焼き

(Pan-fried Chicken Glazed with Soy-mirin Sauce)

Method

1. Heat a non-stick frying pan over a moderate heat until hot.

2. Cook the chicken pieces skin side down. In order to squeeze the fat and excess moisture out of the skin, cook until the skin becomes crisp and golden brown. If the skin is browning too quickly, take the pan off the heat occasionally to slow down the process.

3. When the skin is crisp and golden brown, remove the chicken from the pan, placing it on kitchen paper to drain off any remaining fat. Wipe the frying pan with kitchen paper.

Measurements	Ingredients
4	Large, boned chicken thighs or whole legs with skin
4 tbsp	Cold water
Sauce	
4 tbsp	*Mirin*
1 tbsp	*Sake*
1 ½ tbsp	Japanese soy sauce
1 tsp	Ginger juice made by squeezing freshly grated ginger
Garnish	
1 tbsp	Spring onion, very finely sliced
½ tsp	Grated ginger
1 tsp	Toasted black sesame seeds

4. Return the chicken pieces to the wiped frying pan, cook the flesh side for 1 minute, add cold water and simmer until they are cooked.

5. Combine the *mirin*, *sake* and soy sauce, and pour into the pan.

6. Increase the heat slightly to bring the sauce to the boil. When the sauce becomes syrupy and starts to bubble, add the ginger juice. Keep turning the chicken pieces frequently to coat them in the sauce, taking care not to burn them. Tongs are ideal for this process.

7. When all the chicken pieces are well coated and look glossy, take the pan off the heat. Coat the chicken with the remaining sauce. Garnish with spring onion slices topped with grated ginger at the centre of each chicken piece and sprinkle with toasted black sesame seeds. Serve hot.

Quality Points

- The chicken should look glossy. It should also be succulent with a slightly crunchy skin.

Stir-fried Bean Sprouts, Shiitake Mushrooms and Spring Onions もやしと椎茸の炒めもの

Method

1. Mix the *sake* and soy sauce and set the mixture aside.

2. Heat a wok over a high heat. Add the vegetable oil and swirl it around. Add the garlic and let it sizzle, then add the spring onion. Stir-fry for a few seconds to release the aroma.

3. Add the bean sprouts, and turn and toss them continuously with a spatula over a high heat for about 1 minute, or until the sprouts become slightly opaque but are still crisp. Add the sliced mushrooms and continue to fry for another minute. Sprinkle the water over the vegetables and continue to fry for a further 30 seconds. Pour the *sake* and soy sauce mixture over the vegetables and stir-fry for 30 seconds.

4. Taste and adjust the seasoning with salt and pepper as necessary.

5. Scoop the vegetables onto a serving plate and serve hot.

Measurements	Ingredients
1 tsp	Japanese soy sauce
1 tsp	*Sake*
2 tbsp	Vegetable oil
1 clove	Garlic, crushed and chopped
3	Spring onions, trimmed and cut into 5 cm diagonals
225–350 g	Bean sprouts, with both ends removed
8	Shiitake mushrooms, with stalks removed and cut into 5 mm slices
2 tbsp	Water
	Salt and ground white pepper to taste

Quality Points

- Vegetables should be cooked but crisp, retaining their texture. This dish combines the three vegetables' inherent flavours, enhanced by *sake*, soy and white pepper.

Chef's Tips

- Remove both ends of the bean sprouts for a cleaner taste.

Cucumber and Wakame Seaweed with Japanese Vinegar Dressing

胡瓜とわかめの酢のもの

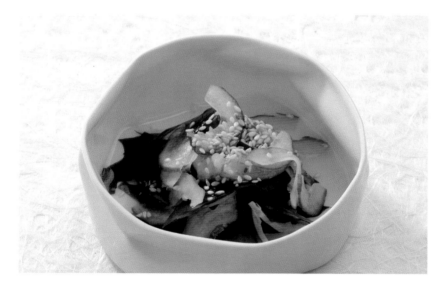

Method

1. Reconstitute the dry *wakame* by soaking it in cold water for 5 minutes. Then blanch in hot water, and plunge into cold water to improve its texture and colour.

2. Trim off any hard ridges and cut into bite-size shapes (5 × 2.5 cm rectangular pieces). Drain.

3. Scoop out the cucumber seeds using a teaspoon. Then slice into paper-thin wedges with a slicer or a mandolin, and soak in the cold salt water for 5 minutes. Drain.

4. Cut the peeled ginger into thin strips and soak them in cold water for 5 minutes to remove any 'too sharp' taste. Drain and pat dry.

5. Combine all the ingredients for the vinaigrette. Mix well and store in the fridge.

6. Just before serving, use half of the vinaigrette to rinse the *wakame*. Drain. Then mix together the cucumber, ginger strips and *wakame*, dressing them in the remainder of the vinaigrette. Distribute them in individual bowls. Sprinkle with crushed white sesame seeds.

Quality Points

- All the vegetables should retain their firm texture. The dressing should have a sweet overtone.

Chef's Tip

- Mix the vegetables with the dressing only just before serving. Do not let them sit in the dressing, as this will make them go soggy and limp.

Measurements	Ingredients
1	Cucumber, cut in half lengthways
50 g	Reconstituted *wakame* seaweed
200 ml	Salt water (1 tsp salt dissolved in 200 ml water)
5 cm	Ginger, peeled
Sanbai-zu vinegar dressing	
100 ml	Japanese rice vinegar
1 ½ tbsp	Caster sugar
½ t sp	Japanese light soy sauce
½ tsp	Salt
Garnish	
1 tsp	Crushed white sesame seeds

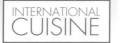
Chicken Broth 鶏の吸いもの

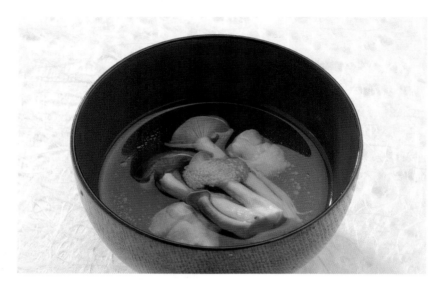

Method

1. Combine all the ingredients for the marinade.

2. Slice the chicken breast into 2.5 cm strips and marinate for 30 minutes.

3. Cut the peeled carrots into thin (2 mm) batons.

4. Break the *shimeji* mushrooms into 3–4 bunches.

5. Take 100 ml of the chicken stock and poach the chicken pieces, carrots and *shimeji* bunches separately until they are just cooked. Drain them on a kitchen towel, cover and leave them aside.

6. Heat the remainder of the chicken stock and the *dashi* stock together and taste; season with salt and light soy sauce.

7. Arrange the poached chicken pieces, carrots and *shimeji* mushrooms artistically in individual soup bowls.

Measurements	Ingredients
Marinade	
1 tsp	*Sake*
Pinch	Salt
Pinch	Ground white pepper
Pinch	Bicarbonate of soda
Pinch	Potato starch
Soup	
50g	Chicken breast
50 g	Carrots, peeled
50 g	*Shimeji* mushrooms
500 ml	Chicken stock (see p. 41)
400 ml	*Dashi* stock (see p. 38)
	Salt
1 tsp	Japanese light soy sauce
Garnish	
2 strips	Lemon peel, cut into very fine julienne (strips)

8. Bring the chicken stock to the boil and ladle it over the soup ingredients, taking care not to spoil the arrangement.

9. Float 2–3 strips of julienne lemon on each bowl. Serve very hot.

Quality Points

* Take care not to overcook the chicken or carrots.

Steamed Rice ご飯

The traditional way of cooking rice is by absorption. The rice is measured by volume rather than weight. The ratio of water to rice is 1:1.

Method

1. Put the rice in a bowl and rinse it under the tap until the water runs almost clear.

2. Soak the washed rice in water for 10 minutes.

3. Place the rice in a sieve, leaving it to drain for 10 minutes.

Measurements	Ingredients
2 cups (400 ml)	Japanese short-grain rice
390 ml	Water (10 ml less than the above formula; see steps 2–4 below)

4. Place the rice in a heavy-bottomed medium-sized pan or a rice cooker and pour in 390 ml of water (this is less water than the standard ratio because of step 2).

5. Put the lid on and bring the rice to the boil over a medium heat, then reduce the heat to a simmer. Cook for a further 5–8 minutes or until all the water has been absorbed and you can hear a crackling noise.

6. Turn off the heat and allow the pan to sit on the stove undisturbed for 5 minutes.

7. Take the lid off the pan and turn the rice over carefully with a rice paddle.

Quality Points

* There should be a sheen on the surface of the cooked rice. The rice should be sticky but firm.

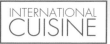

Fish dinner

Grilled Marinated Salmon with Grated *Daikon* Radish 鮭のつけ焼き

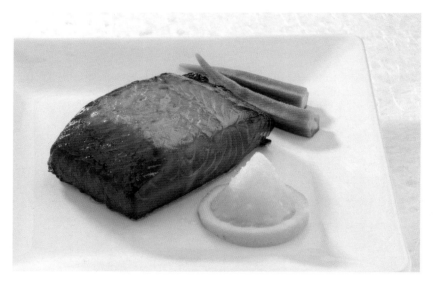

Method

1. Mix the marinade ingredients in a pan and heat slowly to dissolve the sugar completely. Set it aside to cool.

2. Wipe the salmon clean with damp kitchen paper.

3. Marinate the salmon for at least 2 hours. Make sure that the entire surface area of the salmon is covered with the marinade. If not, turn the salmon over several times while marinating.

4. Take out the salmon and wipe off the marinade completely with kitchen paper.

5. Place the fish (skin side up) on a wire rack and cook under a medium grill, taking care not to burn it. The sugar and soy sauce in the marinade will speed up the cooking and make the fish burn easily, so keep a close eye on it.

6. When the salmon is slightly coloured, turn it over to grill the skin side.

7. Arrange the cooked salmon (flesh side up) on individual plates and garnish each with a lemon slice and grated *daikon* radish formed into a pyramid.

Measurements	Ingredients
4 (100–120 g each)	Salmon fillets
Marinade	
125 ml	Japanese soy sauce
125 ml	*Sake*
3 tbsp	Caster sugar
Garnish	
4	Lemon slices
½	*Daikon* radish (mooli), peeled and finely grated

Quality Points

- Fish should be succulent. The outer surface should be crisp and evenly coloured, not burnt.

Chef's Tip

- Swordfish and mackerel work just as well.

Kimpira Carrots
人参のきんぴら

(Stir-fried Sesame-flavoured Julienne Carrots with a Hint of Chilli)

This is a popular Japanese dish. It is traditionally made with carrots and a Japanese vegetable called *gobo* (burdock), which has a crunchy texture and a wonderful earthy flavour, but I have omitted it because it is difficult to get hold of in Europe, and in any case this dish is delicious just with carrots.

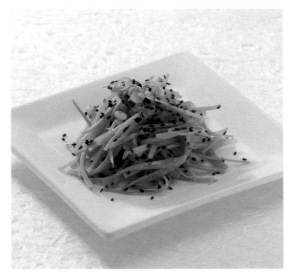

Method

1. Mix the soy sauce, *sake*, rice vinegar and caster sugar and put aside.

2. Heat a wok or frying pan over a high heat. Add the vegetable oil.

3. Fry the chilli until it turns brown, taking care not to burn it. Then discard it.

4. Add the carrots and stir-fry over a high heat for 1 minute. Then add the water to make them wilt. Continue to fry for a further 30 seconds, taking care not to burn the carrots.

5. Add the soy sauce mixture you put aside earlier, coat the carrots with the mixture and stir-fry for a further 30 seconds.

6. Take the wok off the heat, add the sesame oil and mix well.

7. Sprinkle on the crushed sesame seeds.

Measurements	Ingredients
1 tbsp	Japanese soy sauce
1 tbsp	*Sake*
½ tbsp	Japanese rice vinegar
½ tbsp	Caster sugar
1 tbsp	Vegetable oil
1	Dried chilli, deseeded
500 g	Carrots, peeled and cut into 5 cm julienne (strips)
½ tsp	Water
Dash	Sesame oil
2 tbsp	Toasted black sesame seeds, coarsely crushed
Garnish	
1 tbsp	Spring onion, thinly sliced

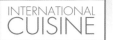
8. Put the carrots in a container and leave to cool.

9. Just before serving, sprinkle on the sliced spring onions.

Quality Points

• Carrots should be cooked but still crunchy, and evenly coloured. They should have a balanced flavour of soy sauce, chilli and sesame.

Chef's Tip

• This dish makes an excellent cold starter for a European meal. It can be made ahead of time (it tastes better after a few hours) and stored for two or three days in the fridge in a plastic container.

Blanched Okra with Japanese Vinegar Dressing オクラの酢のもの

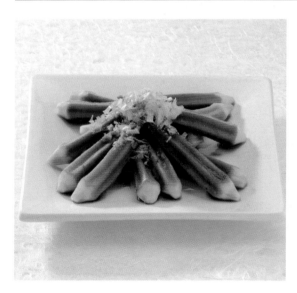

Measurements	Ingredients
200 g	Okra, trimmed and with any dark tips removed
Nihai-zu dressing	
50 ml	Japanese rice vinegar
1 tbsp	Japanese soy sauce
1 tsp	*Mirin*
Garnish	
1 tbsp	Toasted white sesame seeds

Method

1. Blanch the trimmed okra in lightly salted boiling water for 1 minute or until just cooked al dente. Drain and leave it aside to cool.

2. Combine the ingredients for the *nihai-zu* dressing and mix well.

3. Cut each okra diagonally.

4. Arrange the diagonally cut okra on a small plate. Spoon the dressing carefully over the okra and sprinkle on the toasted white sesame seeds.

5. Serve immediately.

Quality Points

- Okra should be slightly crunchy: do not over cook.

Chef's Tip

- Assemble just before serving as the okra will get soggy if left in the dressing for too long. This dish makes a delicious light starter in the summer.

Tofu and Wakame Miso Soup
豆腐とわかめの味噌汁

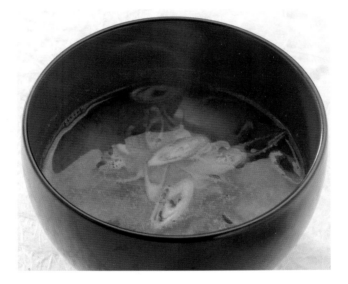

Method

1. Remove all the hard stalks from the *wakame* and cut it into 5 cm lengths.

2. Refresh the tofu by soaking it in warm water for 5 minutes. Then cut it into 1 cm cubes.

3. Place the *dashi* stock and *wakame* in a pan and bring to the boil over a low heat. Add the tofu cubes and simmer until they are heated through.

4. Dissolve the miso with a ladleful of the hot stock and then add to the soup.

Measurements	Ingredients
100–150g	Fresh, firm tofu
25 g	Reconstituted *wakame* seaweed
800 ml	*Dashi* stock
3 heaped tbsp	Miso
Garnish	
2	Spring onions, thinly sliced

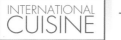

5. Heat to just below boiling point, so as not to spoil the miso's flavour.

6. Serve hot in individual bowls with a sprinkle of sliced spring onion on each.

Quality Points

- The soup should have a good aroma of miso without tasting too salty. Make sure the soup is free of lumps of miso.

Mushroom Rice キノコご飯

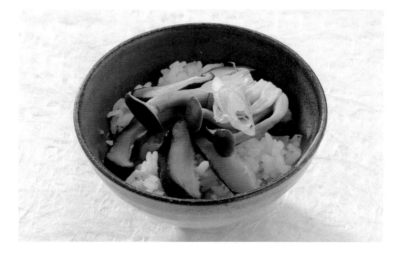

Method

1. Heat the vegetable oil in a non-stick frying pan and add the shiitake mushroom slices. Fry until they are slightly coloured.

2. Put the washed rice in a heavy-bottomed saucepan with a tight lid, or a rice cooker. Mix together the *dashi* stock and soy sauce. Pour this over the rice and put the lid on. Cook following the instructions for steamed rice (p. 79).

3. Turn off the heat, take off the lid and scatter the cooked mushrooms on top of the cooked rice. Put the lid back on and let it rest for 5 minutes.

Measurements	Ingredients
5	Large shiitake mushrooms, cleaned with a damp cloth, stalks removed and cut into 1 mm slices (reserve a few slices to use as garnish)
1 tbsp	Vegetable oil
2 cups (400 ml)	Japanese short-grain rice
Liquid for steaming the rice	
2 cups (400 ml)	*Dashi* stock
1 tbsp	Japanese light soy sauce

4. Just before serving, remove the lid and mix in the mushrooms with a wooden spatula, taking care to mix them in evenly. Serve in individual rice bowls. Arrange a few mushroom slices on top of each portion.

Quality Points

- This dish should have a delicate taste of *dashi* stock and soy sauce.

Chef's Tip

- In addition to shiitake mushrooms, *shimeji* and *enoki* mushrooms can be used.

Tofu dinner

Many people, though aware of tofu's health properties, complain that it is tasteless; you will be pleasantly surprised when you try the following recipe.

Tofu Steak with Japanese Mushrooms and Ginger Sauce 豆腐ステーキ

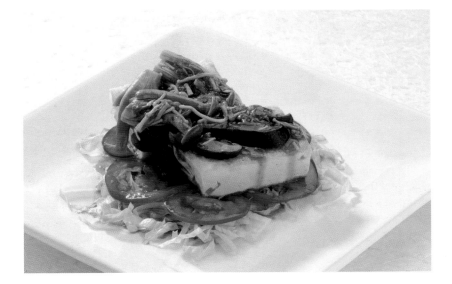

Method

1. Remove the tofu blocks from their plastic packet.

2. To refresh them, rinse in cold water, then steep in warm water for 5 minutes. Pat dry with kitchen paper. In order to squeeze out any excess water, wrap the tofu in a tea towel and put a weight on it for 10 minutes. (A bowl of water on a plate or a block of wood are ideal.)

3. Wipe the mushrooms clean, remove the stalks and cut them into 1 cm slices. Remove the hard ends of the *shimeji* and *enoki*, and divide into bunches of 3–4 stalks each.

4. Cut each tofu block in half (5 × 7.5 cm) and dust with seasoned potato starch. (If using one block of Chinese tofu, cut into 4 pieces).

5. Heat half the vegetable oil in a non-stick frying pan. Sear the tofu pieces over a high heat. Turn them over to sear them golden brown on both sides. Set aside and keep them warm.

6. Pour the remaining vegetable oil into a small saucepan and sauté the ginger and spring onion for 30 seconds over a medium heat. Add the mushrooms you prepared earlier and continue to sauté for another 30 seconds. Then stir in the soy sauce, *sake*, *mirin*, rice vinegar, sugar and water, and bring to the boil. Add the potato starch to thicken and adjust the seasoning if required.

7. Place each piece of tofu on an individual warm plate. Arrange it with the lettuce leaves and tomatoes, and pour the sauce over the tofu. Garnish the centre of each piece of tofu with lemon peel strips. Serve hot.

Measurements	Ingredients
500–600 g	Japanese firm tofu (or 1 block of Chinese tofu)
100 g	Mixed Japanese mushrooms (*shiitake, enoki, shimeji*)
1 tbsp	Potato starch seasoned with salt and ground white pepper
1 tbsp	Vegetable oil
Sauce	
1 tbsp	Ginger, grated
2	Spring onions, finely sliced
2 tbsp	Japanese soy sauce
2 tbsp	*Sake*
1 tbsp	*Mirin*
1 tbsp	Japanese rice vinegar
½ tsp	Caster sugar
2 tbsp	Water
1 tsp	Potato starch (dissolved in 1 tbsp water)
Garnish	
4	Lettuce leaves
1	Tomato, very thinly sliced
1 strip	Lemon peel, cut into fine strips

Quality Points

- Tofu should have a uniformly golden crust.

Stir-fried Boiled Quails' Eggs, Sugar-snap Peas and Spring Onions

うずら卵とえんどうの炒めもの

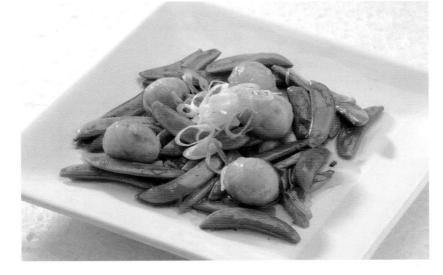

Method

1. Boil the quails' eggs for 5 minutes. Then plunge them in cold water and peel off the shells. Dust with seasoned potato starch, and put aside.

2. Mix the *sake*, sesame oil and soy sauce and set it aside.

3. Heat a wok over a high heat. Pour in half of the vegetable oil and swirl it around to cover the maximum surface area. Add half the garlic, ginger and spring onions, and let them sizzle for 1 minute. Stir to release their aroma.

4. Add the quails' eggs and toss continuously over a high heat, taking care not to burn them. When they are golden, remove the eggs from the wok and set them aside.

Measurements	Ingredients
12	Quails' eggs
1 tbsp	Potato starch, seasoned with salt and ground white pepper
1 tbsp	*Sake*
1 tsp	Sesame oil
1 tbsp	Japanese soy sauce
3 tbsp	Vegetable oil
2 cloves	Garlic, peeled, crushed and chopped
5 cm	Ginger, peeled and cut into very thin strips
3	Spring onions, trimmed
200 g	Sugar-snap peas, trimmed
1 tsp	Potato starch dissolved in 1 tbsp water
	Salt and ground white pepper to taste

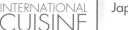

5. Heat the remainder of the vegetable oil in a clean wok and stir-fry the rest of the garlic, ginger and spring onion. Add the sugar-snap peas and the already-cooked garlic, ginger and spring onion, and continue to fry for a further minute.

6. Return the quails' eggs to the wok, pour in the *sake* and soy sauce mixture, and stir well to coat the vegetables and eggs with it.

7. Add the potato starch dissolved in water and mix well. Continue cooking until the sauce is slightly thickened.

8. Adjust the seasoning, adding salt and ground white pepper to taste.

9. Scoop the eggs and vegetables on to a plate and serve hot.

Quality Points

- The sugar-snap peas should be crunchy and the eggs firm. The sauce should be smooth and free of lumps.

Asparagus with Chilli-flavoured Sesame Dressing アスパラガスの胡麻あえ

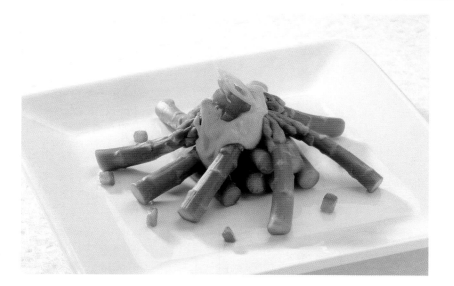

Method

1. Blanch the asparagus in slightly salted water. Remove from the heat while the spears are still crisp and plunge them into cold water to arrest cooking and retain the colour. Cut each spear into two equal lengths.

2. Skin and de-seed the tomatoes and cut them into 1 cm cubes.

3. Prepare the dressing by placing all the ingredients in a bowl and mixing well.

4. Toss the asparagus in half the dressing in a large mixing bowl.

5. Arrange the asparagus spears in a neat pyramid. Garnish the top with tomato cubes.

Quality Points

- The asparagus should be crunchy and succulent. The dressing should taste nutty with a flavour of sesame plus a little heat from the chilli. Tomatoes should give an additional acidity that counterbalances the oil-based dressing.

Chef's Tip

- If the sesame dressing hardens, add a small amount of warm water to loosen it up.

Measurements	Ingredients
20 spears	Asparagus, trimmed and peeled
Dressing	
2 tbsp	*Tahini*
2 tbsp	Japanese rice vinegar
1 tsp	Japanese soy sauce
A few drops	Chinese chilli oil
½ clove	Garlic, crushed into paste
	Salt and ground white pepper to taste
Garnish	
2	Tomatoes, skinned deseeded and cut into 1 cm cubes

Potato and Onion Miso Soup
ジャガイモと玉葱の味噌汁

Method

1. Place the potatoes and onions in a pan full of water and cook over a low heat.

2. Dissolve the miso with a ladleful of hot liquid from the above, and add to the soup.

3. Simmer to bring to the boil and then take the pan off the heat. (The flavour of miso deteriorates when overheated.) Taste to see that the three flavours of potato, onion and miso are harmoniously blended.

4. Serve immediately in individual bowls, garnished with the sliced spring onion.

Measurements	Ingredients
100 g	Potatoes, peeled and cut into 1 cm dice
50 g	Onions, peeled and cut into 1 cm dice
800 ml	Water
3 tbsp	Miso
Garnish	
1 tbsp	Spring onion, very thinly sliced

Quality Points

- The soup should be a blend of slightly salty miso and the natural sweetness of potato and onion. There should be no miso lumps.

Jade Rice 翡翠ご飯

(Seasoned Steamed Rice with Green Peas)

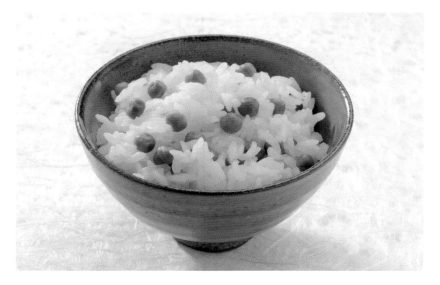

Method

1. Wash the rice as indicated in the steamed rice recipe (see p. 79) and soak it in the 500 ml of water for 30 minutes.

2. Cook the peas in salted boiling water for 2–3 minutes. Drain and retain the liquid.

3. Add 1 cup of the liquid and the seasoning to the rice. Replace the lid and cook.

4. As soon as the rice is cooked, add the peas, put the lid back and leave to stand for 5 minutes.

5. Lift the lid and mix the peas into the rice, taking care not to crush the grains. Transfer to a serving dish and fluff up the rice with a fork before serving.

Measurements	Ingredients
3 cups (600 ml)	Japanese short-grain rice
80 g	Peas (fresh or frozen)
500 ml	Water
Seasoning	
3 tbsp	*Sake*
1 tsp	Salt
1 tsp	Japanese light soy sauce

Quality Points

- As with rice, cooked peas should be al dente.

All recipes serve four, unless stated otherwise.

Sushi Rice

Sushi rice, called *shari* in Japanese, is an essential ingredient of sushi. It is important to use short-grain Japanese rice and to get the right water-to-rice ratio for steaming it. The general rule is an equal volume of water to rice, but for *shari*, taking into account that vinegar is added later, water is reduced by the equivalent amount in order to get the right texture. Sushi rice can be made in advance and stored in a container covered with a clean damp tea towel. A 200 ml cup is used for this recipe.

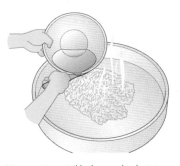

Vinegar is sprinkled over the hot rice (note that the rice is spread over the central part of the dish).

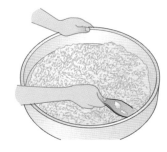

Vinegar is mixed in to the hot rice using a wooden spatula in swift vertical movements

Method

1. Wash rice in a bowl, changing the water a few times until it runs almost clear.

2. Place the rice in a sieve and leave for 5 minutes or until the water has drained off completely.

3. Prepare the sushi vinegar by mixing together the rice vinegar, sugar and salt.

4. Place the rice in a heavy-bottomed medium-sized pan with a tight-fitting lid, or a rice cooker, and pour in the 340 ml of water.

Measurements	Ingredients
2 cups (400 ml)	Japanese short-grain rice
340 ml	Water
Sushi vinegar	
4 tbsp (60 ml)	Japanese rice vinegar
1 ½ tbsp	Caster sugar
½ tsp	Salt

5. Put the lid on the pan and place on a medium heat to bring slowly to the boil. Continue to boil for 2 minutes, then reduce the heat to a simmer and cook for a further 5—8 minutes, or until the water is completely absorbed and you start to hear a crackling noise. It is crucial not to remove the lid.

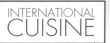
6. Turn off the heat and allow the pan to sit on the stove undisturbed for 1–2 minutes.

7. Remove the lid and turn the rice out into a large bowl. Sprinkle the vinegar mixture over the hot rice and mix it carefully with a wooden spatula, taking care not to crush the grains. To keep the grains separate, use the spatula in a swift vertical motion. Remember to mix in the vinegar as soon as the rice is cooked and piping hot.

8. Spread the rice evenly on a large metal plate or in a wooden sushi tub. Cool to room temperature by fanning. (This gives the rice a sheen and stops it from getting soggy.)

9. When the rice has cooled, it is ready for use.

10. To keep sushi rice from drying out, place it in a container and cover with a clean damp tea cloth. Sushi rice should be eaten on the day it is made. It should not be refrigerated as the rice will harden.

Quality Points

- Sushi rice should be sticky but firm, and taste slightly vinegary with a hint of sweetness.

Sushi Fillings and Toppings 寿司具

Simmered Shiitake Mushrooms 椎茸のうま煮

Preparation

- Reconstitute the dried mushrooms by soaking them in tepid water for an hour, or more if necessary.

Method

1. Squeeze out the excess liquid from the reconstituted mushrooms.

2. Put the mushrooms in a small pan and cover them with water.

3. Simmer for 5 minutes on a very low heat or until the mushrooms are cooked. Add the sugar and simmer for a further 5 minutes.

4. Add the soy sauce and liquid from the reconstituted mushrooms, and continue to simmer until the liquid almost evaporates, taking care not to let the mushrooms stick to the bottom of the pan. Add the *mirin* and cook for 1 minute more to let the alcohol evaporate.

Measurements	Ingredients
6–8	Dried shiitake mushrooms
Seasoning	
100 ml	Water
4 tbsp	Caster sugar
2 tbsp	Japanese soy sauce
1 tbsp	*Mirin*
100 ml	Liquid from the reconstituted mushrooms

5. Remove from the heat. Leave aside until cooled to room temperature.

6. Use as a sushi roll filling or mix with rice for other types of sushi.

Quality Points

- The mushrooms should taste richly sweet with an overtone of soy sauce, look glossy and have a meaty texture.

Chef's Tip

- This dish can be made in advance and frozen or stored in an airtight container for two or three days.

Golden Thread Eggs 錦糸玉子

Method

1. Beat the eggs well with the sugar and salt, making sure the sugar is completely dissolved. Strain.

2. Oil a frying pan. Pour in a small amount of the beaten egg mixture, letting it spread paper thin. Cook over a low heat, taking care not to brown. Turn it over to cook the other side.

Measurements	Ingredients
2	Eggs, beaten
¼ tsp	Caster sugar
¼ tsp	Salt
1 tbsp	Vegetable oil

3. Repeat with the remaining egg mixture. Leave to cool. Cut into 1 mm julienne (strips).

Kanpyo かんぴょう

Method

1. Wash the *kanpyo* and rub it with salt. Reconstitute in lukewarm water. (It will expand to about eight times its size.)

2. Boil for 5 minutes and then drain.

3. Place the boiled *kanpyo* and the *dashi* stock in a pan. Add the sugar and *mirin* and simmer for 10 minutes. Add the soy sauce and cook for a further 5 minutes.

Measurements	Ingredients
25 g	*Kanpyo* (see p. 60)
400 ml	*Dashi* stock
2 tbsp	Caster sugar
1 tbsp	*Mirin*
2 tbsp	Japanese soy sauce

4. Remove from the heat and cool the *kanpyo* in its own juices. Use as required.

Futomaki Rolls 太巻き寿司

Before embarking on this recipe, you may wish to look at the illustrations on pages 95–96, which offer guidance on good technique.

Preparation

- Make sushi rice following the recipe on p. 91.
- Prepare simmered shiitake as shown in the recipe on p. 92.
- Combine the ingredients for the *su-mizu* and put aside. (This is to be used for dampening the hands to prevent the rice sticking.)

Fillings

- Remove the stone from the avocado and cut it into strips 1 cm wide and 12 cm long. Remove the skin and brush the cut pieces with lemon juice to prevent discolouration.
- Rub the cucumber skin with salt until slightly moist. Rinse off the salt completely and pat dry. (This is to remove the raw taste from the skin.) Halve the cucumber lengthways, scoop out the seeds and cut the two halves into batons 0.5 cm wide, 12 cm long.
- Cut the cooked shiitake into 0.5 cm slices.
- Shell and de-vein the prawns.

Method

1. Place a sheet of *nori* shiny side down on a bamboo mat (*maki-su*).
2. Moisten hands with the *su-mizu*. Take a handful of the sushi rice and spread it evenly over the *nori* sheet, leaving a 1 cm gap at the edge on the far side.
3. With your index finger, draw a thin line of *wasabi* across the centre of the rice.

Measurements	Ingredients
4	Standard *nori* sheets
2 cups (400 ml)	Sushi rice
1 tbsp	*Wasabi* powder, mixed with a little water to make a stiff paste
Large pinch	Salt
1	Lemon, juice of
Fillings	
½	Avocado
8	Medium-sized prawns, boiled
50 g	Middle pieces of smoked salmon, cut into 0.5 cm wide, 12 cm long batons (strips)
4	Simmered shiitake mushrooms (see p. 92 for sushi fillings and toppings recipes)
2 tbsp	White sesame seeds, toasted
1	Lebanese cucumber (half a cucumber if the ordinary type is used)
Su-mizu (vinegared water)	
150 ml	Water
1 tbsp	Rice vinegar
Garnish	
4 tbsp (heaped)	Sushi ginger

4. Line up the avocado strips neatly below the *wasabi* line

5. Line up the prawns and cucumber batons, simmered shiitake slices and smoked salmon batons neatly and closely side by side without overlapping.

6. Sprinkle the sesame seeds evenly over the neat rows of fillings.

7. Roll the ingredients in the bamboo mat in the same way you would a roulade, forming a firmly packed cylinder. (See the accompanying photos for guidance on technique.)

8. Use the remaining ingredients to make more rolls.

9. To serve, cut each roll into 4–6 slices. For a clean finish, use a sharp knife and moisten the blade before cutting each slice.

10. Arrange the slices on a plate with the sushi ginger on the side. Serve with a small dish of soy sauce for dipping.

Quality Points

- The roll should be straight and of uniform width. Do not crush the rice grains by packing them in too densely. All the fillings should be at the centre of the roll.

The *futomaki* rolling technique

The photos below show the *futomaki* rolling technique using simmered shiitake, smoked salmon, cucumber and *takuan* radish as fillings.

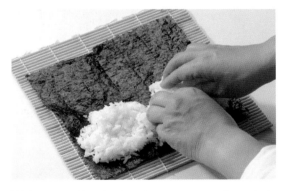

With moistened hands, place the rice on a *nori* sheet which is positioned shiny side down on a bamboo mat (*maki-su*)

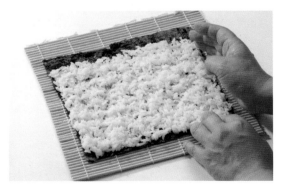

Spread the rice evenly, leaving a 1 cm gap at the edge on the far side

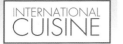

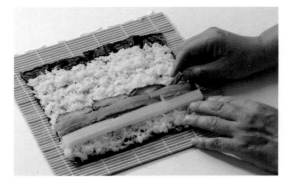

Line up the fillings neatly below a line of *wasabi* at the centre

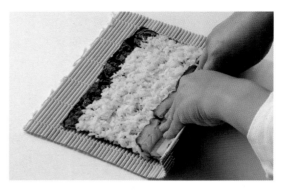

Roll up the ingredients in the bamboo mat, making a firmly packed cylinder

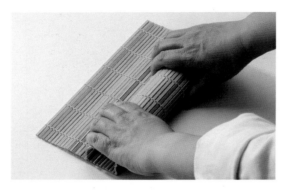

Press the roll into a neat cylinder

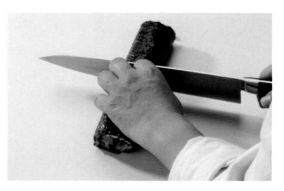

Cut the roll into four to six slices, using a sharp knife, moistening the blade after each slice

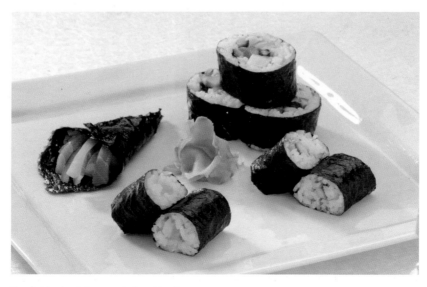

The finished article: assorted sushi rolls

Cucumber Rolls かっぱ巻き

This is a thin roll, ideal for canapés.

Preparation

- Make sushi rice following the recipe on p. 91.
- Mix together the ingredients for the *su-mizu* and put this to one side. (This is to be used for dampening the hands to prevent the rice sticking.)
- Cut the *nori* sheets in half horizontally.

Fillings

- Rub the cucumber skin with salt until slightly moist. Rinse off salt completely and pat it dry. (This is to remove the raw taste from the skin.) Halve the cucumber lengthways, scoop out seeds and cut the two halves into batons 0.5 cm wide, 12 cm long.

Method

(See the photos for *futomaki*, above, for guidance.)

1. Place half a sheet of *nori* shiny side down, on a bamboo mat (*maki-su*).
2. Moisten hands with the *su-mizu*. Take a handful of the sushi rice and spread it evenly over the *nori* sheet, leaving a 1 cm gap at the edge on the far side.
3. With your index finger, draw a thin line of *wasabi* across centre of the rice.
4. Line up the cucumber strips neatly on the *wasabi* line.
5. Sprinkle the sesame seeds evenly over these neat rows of filling.
6. Roll the cucumber strips in the bamboo mat in the same way you would a roulade, forming a firmly packed cylinder (see the photos on pp. 95–96).
7. Use the remaining ingredients to make more rolls.
8. To serve, cut each roll into 6 slices. For a clean cut, use a sharp knife and moisten the blade before each slice.
9. Arrange the slices on a plate with the sushi ginger on the side. Serve with a small dish of soy sauce for dipping.

Quality Points

- The roll should be straight and of uniform width. The rice should not be packed densely so as not to crush the grains. The cucumber should be at the centre of the roll when sliced.

Measurements	Ingredients
1 cup (200 ml)	*Sushi* rice (see p. 91 for recipe)
4–6	Standard *nori* seaweed sheets
4 tbsp	White sesame seeds, toasted
Filling	
1	Lebanese cucumber
Large pinch	Salt
1 tbsp	*Wasabi* powder, mixed with a little water to make a stiff paste
Su-mizu (vinegared water)	
150 ml	Water
1 tbsp	Rice vinegar
Garnish	
2 tbsp (heaped)	Sushi ginger

Chef's Tip

- Substitute with half an ordinary cucumber if the Lebanese variety is unavailable. Other filling suggestions are: fresh tuna, smoked salmon and *takuwan* radish (pickled *daikon* radish).

Temaki Rolls 手巻き寿司

Preparation

- Make sushi rice following the recipe on p. 91.
- Cut the *nori* sheets into quarters.
- Mix the ingredients for the *su-mizu* and put aside. (This is to be used for dampening the hands to prevent the rice sticking.)

Filling

- Cut the avocado lengthways into strips 1 cm wide and 6 cm long. Remove the skin and brush the cut pieces with lemon juice to prevent discolouration.
- Rub the cucumber skin with salt until slightly moist. Rinse off the salt completely and pat dry. (This is to remove the raw taste from the skin.) Halve the cucumber lengthways, scoop out the seeds and cut the two halves into batons 0.5 cm wide, 6 cm long.
- Shell and de-vein the prawns but keep the tails on.
- Cut the cress into equal lengths.
- Arrange the fillings on a large plate.

Method

1. Take a quartered *nori* sheet in your hand, place on it a tablespoonful of sushi rice and then spread on this a bit of *wasabi* paste, using your finger.

2. Place 2–3 strips of the fillings of your choice on top of the rice and *wasabi*, and wrap the *nori* around to form a cone.

3. Eat immediately.

Measurements	Ingredients
1 cup (200 ml)	Sushi rice (see p. 91 for recipe)
Fillings	
1/2	Avocado
8	Medium-sized prawns, boiled
100 g	Middle piece of smoked salmon, cut into batons 0.5 cm wide, 6 cm long
1	Lemon, juice of
8	Standard *nori* sheet
2 tbsp	White sesame seeds, toasted
1	Lebanese cucumber (half a cucumber if the ordinary type is used)
Large pinch	Salt
1 tbsp	*Wasabi* powder, mixed with a little water to make a stiff paste
1 packet	Cress
2	Spring onions, cut into julienne (strips)
Su-mizu (vinegared water)	
150 ml	Water
1 tbsp	Rice vinegar
Garnish	
4 tbsp (heaped)	Sushi ginger

Quality Points

- *Nori* sheets should be crisp, not soggy. Do not stuff with too much rice; work out the best proportion of rice to each filling. These rolls have a refreshing taste.

Chef's Tip

- The rice and fillings can be made a few hours in advance. Keep the rice covered and stored in a cool place; refrigerate the fillings. Let diners make their own rolls at the table.

Nigiri-zushi (Hand-formed Sushi) (にぎりずし)

Method

1. Cut the fish into 1 cm-thick slices, cover and refrigerate.

2. Line up the sushi rice, a bowl of vinegared water, *wasabi* paste, the fish slices and a serving platter.

3. Dip the fingers of both hands in the vinegared water. Dampen the palms too.

4. Lift about a tablespoonful of sushi rice with your right hand, gently pressing and forming it into a boat shape (see the diagrams of steps 1 and 2 on p. 100).

Measurements	Ingredients
2 cups	Prepared sushi rice (see p. 91 for recipe)
200 g	Uncut tuna fillet, a 6/7 cm × 3 cm block
150 ml	Vinegared water (see p. 94)
2 tbsp	Prepared *wasabi* paste
3 tbsp	Sushi ginger

5. Lift a slice of fish with the index finger and thumb of the left hand. Holding the rice 'boat' in the fist of your right hand, use the tip of your right-hand index finger to scoop up a dab of *wasabi*. Spread the *wasabi* in the middle of the slice of fish (see the diagrams of steps 3 and 4).

6. Bend the fingers of the left hand to form a cup to hold the fish; place the boat-shaped rice on to the centre of the slice of fish. (The fish slice is usually longer and wider than the rice boat.) (See the diagram of step 5).

7. Using the right-hand index and middle fingers, gently press the rice boat and fish together (see the diagram of step 6).

8. Gently flip over the sushi so that the fish is on top. Tidy up the edges, thus making the sushi presentable (see the diagrams of steps 7–9).

9. Press the sushi again with the right-hand index and middle fingers (see the diagram of step 10).

10. Arrange on a serving platter with the sushi ginger.

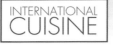

Making Nigiri-zushi

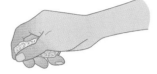

Step 1: Press the sushi rice in your right hand

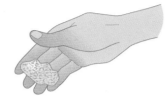

Step 2: Form the rice into a 'boat' shape

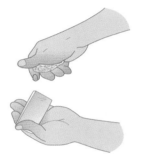

Step 3: Holding a slice of fish in the left hand, place a dab of *wasabi* on the right index finger (the rice is still held in the right hand)

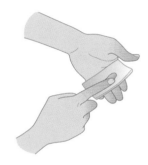

Step 4: Spread the *wasabi* on the slice of fish

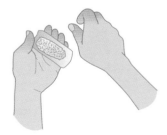

Step 5: Place the rice on to the centre of the slice of fish

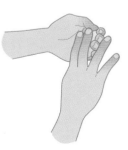

Step 6: Press the rice 'boat' and the fish together

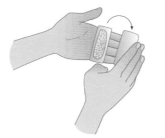

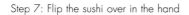

Step 7: Flip the sushi over in the hand

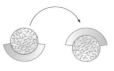

Step 8: Flipping the sushi

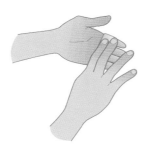

Step 9: Tidy up the edges

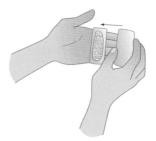

Step 10: Press the sushi again, to finish

Fukusa-zushi and Chakin-zushi

ふくさ寿司 と 茶巾寿司

These two are the same basic sushi recipe presented in different ways.

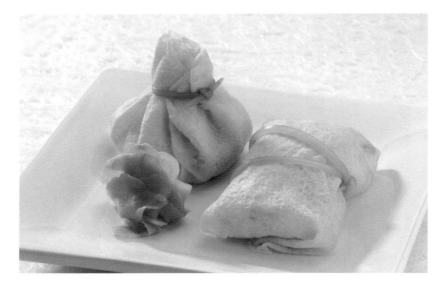

Method: Fukusa-zushi

1. Combine the beaten eggs with the sugar and salt and mix well. Strain the liquid.

2. Heat a small non-stick frying pan. Lightly oil the surface and use enough of the egg mixture to make a very thin flat omelette. Do not allow the egg to colour. Repeat the process to make as many omelettes as possible with the remaining egg mixture. Leave the omelettes to cool. (Do not stack them as they will stick together.)

3. Mix the mushroom slices and toasted sesame seeds into the sushi rice.

4. Cut the edges off each omelette to make them square.

5. Place a square omelette on a clean flat surface. Turn the omelette through 45° so it forms a diamond shape.

Measurements	Ingredients
2 cups (400 ml)	Sushi rice (see p. 91 for recipe)
8	Simmered shiitake mushrooms (see the sushi filling and topping recipes on p. 92), thinly sliced
2 tbsp	Lightly toasted white sesame seeds
8	Long, flat parsley stalks, blanched and with the leaves removed
1 tbsp	Vegetable oil
Omelette mix	
2	Eggs, well beaten
¼ tsp	Sugar
¼ tsp	Salt
Garnish	
2 tbsp	Sushi ginger

6. Place 1 ½ tablespoonsful of sushi rice in the middle of the omelette and fold the corner nearest to you over the filling.

7. Then fold the left and right corners on top.

8. Turn the omelette over to the top corner to make a rectangular parcel.

9. Tie the parcel neatly using the blanched parsley stalks.

10. Repeat the process with the remaining omelettes and rice.

11. Arrange one or two parcels per portion on a plate and garnish with the sushi ginger.

Method: Chakin-zushi

1. Follow the *fukusa-zushi* recipe above, up to step 3.

2. Place an omelette on a clean flat surface.

3. Place 1 ½ tablespoonsful of the sushi rice in the middle.

4. Gather up the edges of the omelette neatly to make a 'money bag' and tie with blanched parsley stalks.

5. Serve as in step 11 of *fukusa-zushi*.

Chef's Tip

• These are excellent ways of using up leftover sushi rice.

Inari-zushi いなり寿司

(Stuffed Sushi Rice in Seasoned Fried Tofu Pouches)

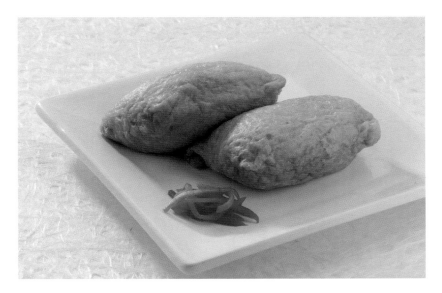

Preparation

- Make the sushi rice following the recipe on p. 91. Mix in the filling ingredients thoroughly.

- Combine the water and rice vinegar to make *su-mizu* and put aside. (This is to be used for dampening the hands when stuffing in the rice.)

Method

1. Place a sheet of *age* on a clean chopping board and roll a chopstick up and down its length. (Think of it as a mini rolling pin.) This separates the two sides of the *age* and forms an 'envelope'. Cut this in half crosswise and carefully open up each half into a pouch.

2. Put these pouches into boiling water and boil for 1–2 minutes to remove oil.

3. Drain and squeeze out the excess water gently.

4. Put the pouches in a pan and cover them with the *dashi* stock and sugar, and bring to the boil. Reduce the heat to a simmer and cook for 2–3 minutes. Then add the soy sauce and continue to simmer until the liquid is reduced to one-third. Cool the pouches in this liquid.

5. Take each pouch and squeeze out any excess liquid gently. Open the pouch carefully and fill it with *sushi* rice, taking care not to over-fill. Once it is full, fold over the open edges and tuck them underneath.

6. Arrange 2–3 pouches per portion on a plate and garnish with the *beni-shoga* (red salted ginger) julienne on the side.

Measurements	Ingredients
2 cups (400 ml)	Sushi rice
8 sheets	*Age* (Japanese fried bean curd)
Filling	
3 tbsp	Toasted white sesame seeds
6	Shiitake mushrooms, simmered and chopped very finely
1	Lemon, rind of, very finely chopped
Seasoning	
200 ml	*Dashi* stock
1 tbsp	Caster sugar
1 tbsp	Japanese soy sauce
Su-mizu (vinegared water)	
150 ml	Water
1 tbsp	Rice vinegar
Garnish	
3 tbsp	*Beni-shoga* (red-coloured salted ginger), cut into julienne

Quality Points

- Sushi should taste slightly sweet when eaten from the pouch, with a hint of vinegar from the sushi rice.

Chef's Tip

- It is vital to add the sugar first, before the soy sauce, otherwise the pouches will get salty. They can be made in advance and frozen.

Braised Beef and Tofu in Sweet Miso
牛肉と豆腐の炊き合わせ

Preparation

- Wrap the tofu in a tea towel and place a weight on it to squeeze out any excess water.

- Sprinkle salt over the *konnyaku* and pound on it a few times with a rolling pin. Wash off the salt in warm water. Tear or cut the *konnyaku* into bite-size pieces and dry-toast them in a pan to evaporate any excess moisture.

Method

1. Trim the beef and slice very thinly (1 cm) and cut into bite-size pieces. Blanch these in hot water and drain.

2. Cut the tofu into 2 cm cubes.

3. Place the beef, *konnyaku*, water and *sake* in a pan, cover with a drop-lid (see p. 25) and simmer for 1 hour. Skim frequently.

4. When the meat is tender, add the brown sugar, miso, garlic and ginger, and cook for a further 30 minutes with a drop-lid on. Taste, and adjust the seasoning if required.

5. Add the spring onion and tofu, and cook gently until the tofu cubes are heated through.

6. Transfer into individual bowls and serve hot with mustard and *shichimi* chilli on the side as condiments.

Quality Points

- The beef should be tender but the other ingredients should be al dente. The sauce should have a sweet miso flavour.

Measurements	Ingredients
500 g	Beef rib or brisket
100 g	Japanese or Chinese firm tofu
1 sheet	*Konnyaku*
2	Garlic cloves, finely chopped
5 cm	Ginger, finely chopped
4	Spring onions (white part only), cut into 2 cm lengths
Stock	
600 ml	Water
200 ml	*Sake*
30 g	Brown sugar
50 g	Miso
Condiments	
1 tbsp	Freshly prepared English mustard
¼ tsp	*Shichimi* pepper

Chef's Tip

- This dish tastes better if cooked in advance. *Konnyaku* can be substituted with peeled and bevelled potatoes or *daikon* radish (mooli) if necessary. Be sure to blanch them first.

Braised Hijiki Seaweed and Fried Bean Curd ひじきと油揚げの炊き合わせ

Preparation

- Reconstitute the *hijiki* seaweed by soaking it in a large bowl of water for 20 minutes. When it expands and becomes soft, wash in cold water to remove any sand. Leave it in a sieve to drain.

- Blanch the *age* sheets in boiling water to remove surface oil. Cut them in half lengthways and then cut into 1 cm-wide strips.

Method

1. Heat the oil in a pan and swiftly stir-fry the *hijiki*. Add the sliced *age* and continue to fry for a further 2 minutes.

2. Add the water, bring to the boil then add the sugar and cook for another minute. Add the soy sauce, reduce the heat to a simmer and continue to cook until the liquid is absorbed.

3. Finally, add the *mirin*, adjust the seasoning and leave to cool. It should taste slightly sweet.

4. Sprinkle on the toasted sesame seeds as garnish and serve in individual small bowls at room temperature.

Measurements	Ingredients
1 tbsp	Vegetable oil
25 g	Dried *hijiki* seaweed
2 sheets	*Age* (fried bean curd)
100 ml	Water
2 tbsp	Caster sugar
2 tbsp	Japanese soy sauce
1 tsp	*Mirin*
	Salt and ground white pepper to taste
Garnish	
1 tbsp	Toasted white sesame seeds

Quality Points

- *Hijiki* seaweed should have a firm texture and a slightly sweet soy flavour.

Chef's Tip

- This is a dish for enjoying the texture of the seaweed. A perfect accompaniment to steamed rice, it tastes better if made in advance.

Chilled Tofu Squares 冷奴

This is a delicious dish on a hot summer's day.

Method

1. Cut the tofu into 5 cm squares.

2. Place the tofu cubes in a large glass bowl and fill it with cold water until the tofu is covered. Then float the cucumber slices and ice cubes on the top.

3. Place each of the condiments on a separate dish.

4. Serve the chilled tofu with a small plate of soy sauce for each diner, thus allowing the addition of sauce and condiments according to individual taste.

Chef's Tip

- Make sure the tofu is very fresh. If the silken type is not available, use the cotton variety.

Measurements	Ingredients
500–600 g	Japanese silken tofu
	Cold water
Garnish	
	Ice cubes
5 cm	Cucumber, very thinly sliced
Condiments	
4	Spring onions, very finely chopped
2.5 cm	Ginger, finely grated
10	*Shiso* leaves (green perilla), finely shredded
	Japanese soy sauce to serve

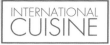
Deep-fried Tofu Squares with Dashi Sauce

揚げだし豆腐

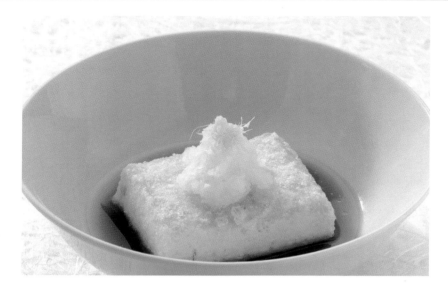

Preparation

- Wrap the tofu in a tea towel and place a clean chopping board or similar on top to add weight. Leave for up to an hour to squeeze out the excess water. Cut into 5 cm squares.

Method

1. Place all the ingredients for the sauce in a pan and bring to the boil to evaporate the alcohol in the *mirin*. Taste, and adjust the seasoning if necessary.

2. Coat each tofu cube lightly with the seasoned potato starch.

3. Deep-fry 2 to 3 cubes at a time for about 6–8 minutes, until they are golden and crispy.

4. Drain the fried tofu squares on absorbent kitchen paper and keep them hot.

5. Keep the oil clean by skimming off any leftover particles.

Measurements	Ingredients
500–600 g	Fresh, firm Japanese or Chinese tofu
2–3 tbsp	Potato starch seasoned with salt and ground white pepper
	Vegetable oil for deep-frying
Sauce	
200 ml	*Dashi* stock
1 tbsp	Japanese soy sauce
2 tbsp	*Mirin*
Garnish	
4 tbsp	Freshly grated *daikon* radish (mooli)
2 tsp	Grated ginger
4	*Shiso* leaves (green perilla), finely shredded

6. Transfer the hot tofu cubes to individual bowls. Reheat the sauce and pour it around the tofu. Garnish with the grated *daikon* radish topped with grated ginger. Serve immediately.

Quality Points

- The tofu should be fluffy and moist inside and crisp on the outside. The sauce should be hot and have a hint of sweetness.

Chef's Tip

- This makes a good starter.

Grilled Tofu Squares with Dengaku Miso Sauce 豆腐の田楽

Preparation

- Wrap the tofu in a tea towel and leave under a weight for 20 minutes to drain off the excess moisture,

- Soak the dried prawns in the *sake* until they are soft, and chop them finely.

- Prepare the garnish by mixing together the thinly sliced spring onions and the shredded *shiso* leaves.

Method

1. Heat the sesame oil and vegetable oil together in a pan, sauté the chopped prawns, shallots and ginger over a low heat until they are soft. Add all the ingredients for the *dengaku* miso, and stir constantly over a low heat until the sauce thickens.

2. Taste the sauce to check it is slightly sweet. If it is salty, add a pinch more sugar.

3. Cut the tofu into 5 cm squares and dry the cut surfaces with paper towels. Brush each cube with vegetable oil and grill them until they are crisp and golden.

4. To serve, spread the *dengaku* miso sauce on the centre of individual serving plates. Mount hot tofu cubes on top and then spoon the miso sauce over them. Garnish with the spring onion slices and *shiso* leaves. Serve hot.

Measurements	Ingredients
500–600 g	Japanese or Chinese firm tofu
30 g	Dried prawns
2 tbsp	*Sake* (for soaking the dried prawns)
1 tbsp	Sesame oil
1 tbsp	Vegetable oil
50 g	Shallots, very finely chopped
5 cm	Ginger, very finely chopped
	Vegetable oil for grilling
Dengaku miso sauce	
150 g	*Akadashi* miso
50 g	White miso
2	Egg yolks
2 tbsp	Caster sugar
4 tbsp	Sake
Garnish	
4	Spring onions (green part only), very thinly sliced
4	*Shiso* leaves (green perilla), finely shredded

Quality Points

- Tofu should be crispy on the outside and soft inside. The sauce should be sweet with a hint of ginger and prawn.

Chef's Tip

- This delicious dish makes an excellent starter.

Simmered Tofu Squares 湯豆腐

You will need an earthenware casserole dish, or pot with a lid, and a tabletop burner.

Method

1. Wipe both sides of the *konbu* with a damp cloth to remove any dirt. Do not wash the *konbu*.

2. Cut the tofu into 5 cm squares.

3. Put each of the condiments on a separate plate.

4. Fill the casserole dish or pot with cold water and add the *konbu*. Leave to stand for 20–30 minutes.

5. Put the pot on a tabletop burner and bring to the boil over a low heat.

Measurements	Ingredients
500–600 g	Japanese firm tofu
20 cm square	Dried *konbu*
Condiments	
4	Spring onions, finely chopped
5 cm	Ginger, finely grated
30 g	*Hana-gatsuo* (bonito flakes)
	Japanese soy sauce to taste

6. Add some of the tofu squares and bring to the boil on a low heat, taking care not to overcook. As tofu overcooks easily it is better to add a few pieces at a time.

7. Serve the tofu piping hot with a small plate of soy sauce for each diner, thus allowing the addition of sauce and condiments according to individual taste.

Vegetables in Tofu and White Miso Sauce 野菜の白あえ

Preparation

- **Dried shiitake mushrooms:** Reconstitute the dried mushrooms by soaking them in lukewarm water with a pinch of sugar. When they are soft, remove the stalks, cut them into julienne (strips) and squeeze them to remove excess moisture. Mix the water, sugar and mushrooms in a pan, bring to the boil and simmer for 3 minutes, taking care not to let them burn. Add the soy sauce and continue to simmer for another minute, and finally add the *mirin*. Cook until the liquid is absorbed and then put aside to cool.

- **Tofu:** Wrap the tofu in dry tea towels and place a clean chopping board or similar on top to add weight. Leave for 30 minutes to squeeze out excess water.

- **Carrots and *daikon* radish (mooli):** Sprinkle salt over the *daikon* and mix well. When it has wilted slightly, rinse off the salt in cold water. Squeeze well to remove any excess moisture.

- **Konnyaku:** Sprinkle salt over the *konnyaku* and pound on it a few times with a rolling pin to soften. Rinse off the salt in cold water and then in boiling water. Cut it into 5 cm julienne and dry-toast in a pan until the excess moisture evaporates. Leave to one side.

Method

1. To make the sauce, add the warm water to the *tahini* and soy sauce, and emulsify in a food processor to make a smooth liquid. Add the tofu and keep processing until it turns into a smooth paste. Combine this with the white miso, *mirin*, sugar and salt. Finally add a few drops of the chilli oil.

2. Add the *daikon* radish, carrots, mushrooms and *konnyaku* to the sauce and serve in individual bowls garnished with the shredded *shiso* (green perilla) and sprinkled with sesame seeds.

3. Serve at room temperature.

Quality Points

- The sauce should be smooth and slightly sweet with a hint of chilli and sesame flavour.

Chef's Tip

- All preparation, including the sauce, can be done in advance. Assemble just before serving.

Measurements	Ingredients
8	Dried shiitake mushrooms
30 g	Carrots, peeled and cut into 5 cm-long julienne (strips)
80 g	*Daikon* radish (mooli), peeled and cut into 5 cm-long julienne (strips)
½ cake	*Konnyaku*
For simmering the shiitake mushrooms	
4 tbsp	Water
2 tbsp	Caster sugar
2 tbsp	Japanese soy sauce
½ tbsp	*Mirin*
Sauce	
1 tbsp	Warm water
2 tbsp	*Tahini* paste
2 tsp	Japanese soy sauce
100 g	Tofu
40 g	White miso
2 tsp	*Mirin*
2 tsp	Caster sugar
Pinch	Salt
2–3 drops	Chinese chilli oil
Garnish	
4	*Shiso* (green perilla) leaves, finely shredded
1 tbsp	Toasted white sesame seeds

Avocado with Wasabi Dressing
アヴォカドのわさび醤油あえ

Preparation

- Make up the *wasabi* paste by mixing 1 tbsp *wasabi* powder with 2 tsp water to make a stiff paste. Cover the paste and put it aside for 1–2 minutes to make it pungent.

Method

1. Cut the avocados in half lengthways. Pull them apart and remove the stones. Peel and cut the flesh into 3 cm cubes. Toss them in the lemon juice.

2. To make the dressing, dissolve the prepared *wasabi* paste in the soy sauce. Add the rest of the dressing ingredients and mix well, making sure there are no *wasabi* lumps.

3. Coat the avocado cubes with the dressing.

4. Arrange the tomato slices concentricallly on each serving plate and pile avocado cubes in the middle with the tomato cubes at the apex. Serve as part of a Japanese set meal or as a starter in a European-style meal

Measurements	Ingredients
2	Ripe avocados
1	Lemon, juice of
Dressing	
½ tsp	*Wasabi* paste
1 tbsp	Japanese soy sauce
1 tbsp	Japanese rice vinegar
½ tbsp	*Sake*
Garnish	
2 tbsp	Skinned and seeded tomato cubes
4	Plum tomatoes, skinned and cut into 1 mm slices

Quality Points

- The avocado should be soft but not mushy. The dressing should taste neither bitter nor sharp.

Chef's Tip

- *Wasabi* powder is preferable to *wasabi* paste in a tube for consistency of taste. Dress the avocado just before serving to prevent it getting mushy. Alternatively, it can be sliced and arranged into a fan for serving.

Aubergine Dengaku 茄子の田楽

(Shallow-fried Aubergines with Dengaku Miso Sauce)

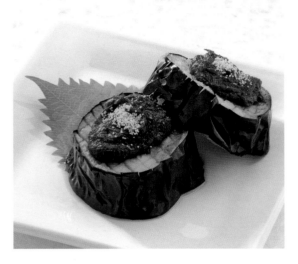

Measurements	Ingredients
2 large	Aubergines
4 tbsp	Vegetable oil
Miso sauce	
1 tbsp	Sesame oil
150 g	*Akadashi* miso
50 g	White miso
2	Egg yolks
4 tbsp	Caster sugar
100 ml	*Sake*
1 tsp	Freshly squeezed ginger juice
Garnish	
1 tbsp	White poppy seeds

Method

1. Remove and discard the stems from the aubergines, and cut into 5 cm-thick rounds. Score the flesh in a lattice pattern on one side of each round.

2. Heat the oil in a frying pan and shallow fry the aubergine slices until golden, especially on the scored side. Drain on kitchen paper, leave aside and keep warm.

3. Heat the sesame oil in a small pan, add all the ingredients for the sauce except the ginger juice, and continue to stir over a medium heat until the sauce thickens to the consistency of peanut butter. Remove from the heat and add the ginger juice. Mix well.

4. Place the fried aubergine slices, scored side up, on a plate and spoon over the sauce. Garnish the centre with white poppy seeds. Serve hot.

Quality Points

• Aubergine slices should not be oily. The sauce should have the aroma of miso, ginger and a hint of sesame.

Chef's Tip

• Surplus miso sauce can be stored in an airtight container and refrigerated for later use.

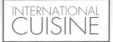

Blanched Spinach Seasoned with Mustard-flavoured Soy Sauce ほうれん草の辛子醤油あえ

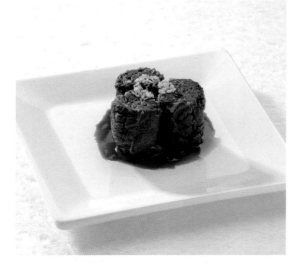

Measurements	Ingredients
400 g	Spinach
Sauce	
½ tsp	Freshly prepared English mustard
2 tbsp	Japanese soy sauce
½ tbsp	Water
1–2 drops	Sesame oil
Garnish	
1 tbsp	Toasted white sesame seeds

Method

1. Cook the spinach in a covered dry pan over a medium heat for 1 minute. Remove the lid and stir the spinach to make it wilt.

2. Remove from the heat and plunge the spinach into a bowl of cold water to arrest cooking.

3. Drain the cooled spinach in a colander and, by hand, squeeze out the bitter juice and excess moisture as much as possible. The spinach should end up looking like a tight ball.

4. Cut the spinach in equal 5 cm lengths.

5. Dissolve the mustard completely in the soy sauce and water mixture. Add a few drops of sesame oil.

6. Coat the spinach in the mustard sauce and mix well.

7. Serve the spinach on small individual plates and pour on any remaining sauce. Garnish with the white sesame seeds at the centre.

Quality Points

• Make sure the spinach is cooked al dente so that it has bite to it. The sauce should have a balanced taste of mustard and soy sauce with a hint of sesame.

Chef's Tip

- It is possible to make a roulade with the spinach: serve sliced, garnishing the cut surface with white sesame seeds. Watercress works well with this recipe, instead of spinach.

Chicken and Cucumber in Japanese Vinegar Dressing きゅうりと鶏肉の酢の物

Method

1. Rub the chicken with *sake* and leave for 10 minutes. Then sprinkle with the salt and sugar, and steam for 20 minutes.

2. Chill the cooked chicken. When cool enough to handle, tear by hand into thin strips.

3. Rub the cucumbers with salt to remove any raw flavour and rinse with cold water. Cut lengthways and remove the seeds. Slice very thinly using a slicer, and sprinkle with a pinch of salt.

4. Squeeze the cucumber slices hard to remove excess water, mix with a small amount of the *sanbai-zu* dressing and squeeze again.

5. To serve, combine the cucumber slices and chicken strips and coat with the *sanbai-zu* dressing. Arrange on individual dishes, pour on the remaining dressing and garnish with ginger strips.

Measurements	Ingredients
300 g	Boned chicken breasts with skin left on
2 tbsp	*Sake*
½ tsp	Salt
¼ tsp	Caster sugar
6	Lebanese cucumbers
200 ml	*Sanbai-zu* dressing (see p. 42 for recipe)
Garnish	
5 cm	Ginger, cut into 1–2 mm strips, soaked in cold water for 30 minutes

Quality Points

- The chicken and cucumber should have a good texture, and be well coated with dressing without being soggy.

Chef's Tip

- This dish offers an economical way of using up cooked chicken. To prevent the chicken getting soggy, dress it just before serving. Try to use Lebanese cucumbers instead of the usual European variety, as they have more flavour.

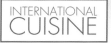
Chinese Leaves and Spinach Roll with Ground Sesame Soy Sauce

白菜とほうれん草のごま醤油

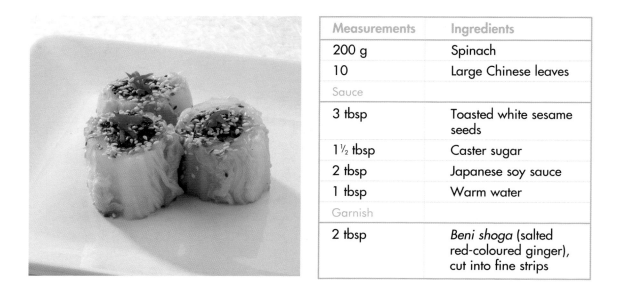

Measurements	Ingredients
200 g	Spinach
10	Large Chinese leaves
Sauce	
3 tbsp	Toasted white sesame seeds
1½ tbsp	Caster sugar
2 tbsp	Japanese soy sauce
1 tbsp	Warm water
Garnish	
2 tbsp	*Beni shoga* (salted red-coloured ginger), cut into fine strips

Preparation

- Wash the spinach thoroughly to remove any dirt, and discard any yellowed leaves and tough stalks.
- Wash the Chinese leaves and trim the ends for a tidy appearance.

Method

1. Cook the spinach in a covered dry pan over a medium heat for 1 minute. Remove the lid and stir the spinach to make it wilt.

2. Remove from the heat and plunge the spinach into a bowl of cold water to arrest cooking.

3. Drain the cold spinach in a colander. Squeeze out the bitter juice and excess moisture as much as possible, using both hands, leaving it looking like a ball. Leave aside.

4. Blanch the Chinese leaves in 100 ml boiling water and drain in a colander. Sprinkle with salt and leave to cool. Squeeze out any excess moisture.

5. Make a roulade by spreading cling film flat on a surface, one piece of the film slightly overlapping another to form a large rectangle.

6. Spread the Chinese leaves horizontally and uniformly on the cling film, leaving at least a 2.5 cm gap at the top and bottom of the film. Place the spinach at the centre to form the core of the cabbage roll.

7. Starting at the near side, roll the Chinese leaves over the spinach, pressing down to push out any trapped air. Keep rolling, making sure that there is no cling film caught in the roulade.

8. Using a sharp knife, cut the roulade into 5 cm-thick rounds and remove the cling film.

9. Food-process or grind the toasted white sesame seeds with a pestle and mortar until they turn into a coarse paste. Add the sugar, soy sauce and warm water, and mix well.

10. Spread the sauce on a plate and place the roulade slices on top. Garnish with the red-coloured *beni shoga* at the centre of each slice.

Quality Points

- Chinese leaves and spinach should be cooked al dente. Each roulade slice should have the green spinach at the centre surrounded by white and opaque Chinese leaves.

Chef's Tip

- It helps to squeeze out as much excess water from the spinach and Chinese leaves as possible before making a roulade. *Tahini* paste is a useful substitute for ground sesame seeds.

French Beans with Crushed Sesame Seeds
インゲンの生姜醤油あえ

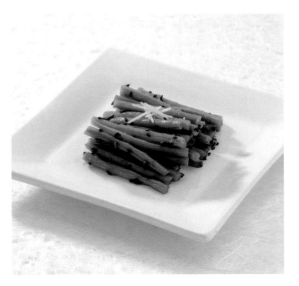

Measurements	Ingredients
200 g	Trimmed fine French beans, cut into 3 cm lengths
Dressing	
2 tbsp	Grated ginger
2 tbsp	Japanese soy sauce
1 tbsp	*Mirin*
Garnish	
1 tsp	Ginger, finely shredded
½ tsp	Toasted black sesame seeds

Method

1. Cook the beans for 2–3 minutes in salted boiling water. Drain and plunge them in cold water to prevent further cooking and discolouration. Drain again when cool.

2. Combine all the ingredients for the dressing, mix well and strain to remove any bits of ginger fibre.

3. Mix the beans with the dressing, letting them absorb the flavour.

4. To serve, pile the beans neatly on a serving plate and garnish with shredded ginger at the apex. Sprinkle the toasted sesame seeds on top.

Quality Points

- French beans should be cooked al dente. The sauce should have a balanced flavour of ginger and soy sauce with a slightly sweet overtone.

Chef's Tip

- Any green beans can be substituted for French beans.

Simmered Bamboo Shoots and Wakame Seaweed 若竹煮

Method

1. Cut the bamboo shoots into equal 5 cm chunks.

2. Reconstitute the dried *wakame* seaweed in cold water and remove any hard stalks. Cut into 2.5 cm squares.

3. Place the shoots and 600 ml of the *dashi* stock in a pan and bring to the boil.

4. Reduce the heat to a simmer and add the sugar, salt and light soy sauce. Continue to cook for about 30 minutes.

5. Add the remaining 400 ml of *dashi* stock to the bamboo shoots and continue to simmer.

6. Squeeze the *wakame* squares, add to the bamboo and simmer for 2 minutes.

7. Remove from the heat.

8. Arrange the bamboo shoots neatly in individual bowls with the *wakame* at the centre of each. Keep warm.

Measurements	Ingredients
500 g	Cooked bamboo shoots
40 g	Reconstituted *wakame* seaweed
Stock	
1 litre	*Dashi* stock
2½ tbsp	Caster sugar
¼ tbsp	Salt
1½ tbsp	Japanese light soy sauce
½ tsp	Potato starch mixed with 1 tsp water
Pinch	Ground *sansho* pepper
20	*Kinome* leaves (optional)

9. Reheat the stock, adding the potato starch mixture to thicken it very slightly, and mix in the *sansho* pepper.

10. Spoon the hot stock on to the arranged bamboo shoots, and serve hot. Garnish with *kinome* leaves if desired.

Quality Points

- Bamboo shoots and *wakame* leaves should have an al dente texture.

Chef's Tip

- Since *kinome* leaves are difficult to find, ground *sansho* pepper is used to add tanginess to the dish.

Simmered Daikon Radish with Miso Sauce
ふろふき大根

Method

1. Peel the *daikon* radish and cut it into four 5 cm slices, bevelling the edges (see p. 29). Make criss-cross incisions on one side only.

2. Place the *daikon* slices in a pan and add enough water to cover them.

3. Add the *konbu* and sprinkle in the rice. Bring to the boil over a high heat.

4. Reduce to a low heat and leave to simmer.

5. After 5 minutes, remove the *konbu* from the pan and continue to simmer for about 20 minutes, or until the radish becomes soft and translucent.

6. Turn off the heat and leave aside.

7. Pour all the sauce ingredients into another pan. Mix well and bring slowly to the boil.

8. Reduce the heat to a simmer and stir continuously until the sauce thickens.

Measurements	Ingredients
20 cm	*Daikon* radish (mooli)
10 cm square	Dried *konbu*
2 tbsp	White rice
Miso sauce	
40 g	White miso
70 g	*Shinshu* miso
100 ml	*Dashi* stock
1 tbsp	*Mirin*
4 tbsp	Caster sugar
Garnish	
½ tsp	Grated *yuzu* rind (use tangerine if *yuzu* is unavailable)

9. Arrange one hot simmered *daikon* slice in the centre of each plate and spoon the miso sauce over the top, then sprinkle on the grated *yuzu* rind. Serve hot.

Quality Points

- The *daikon* should be soft but not bitter. The miso sauce should be highly aromatic with a hint of citrus fragrance.

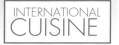
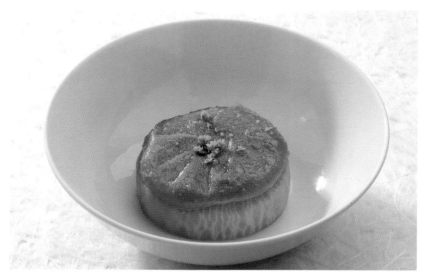

Chef's Tip

- Do not forget the rice – it removes the bitterness of the *daikon* and prevents it darkening when cooked.

Simmered Kabocha Squash かぼちゃの煮つけ

This is a typical autumn dish when *kabocha* squash is in season. For a successful result, follow the simmering technique described on p. 25.

Method

1. Cut the *kabocha* squash in half and remove the seeds.

2. Cut it into 6–7 cm rectangular pieces and bevel the edges (see p. 29).

3. Partially remove the skin in alternate strips.

4. Place the *kabocha* pieces, skin side down, in a pan.

5. Add the water, sugar and *sake* together to the pan, so that the *kabocha* is just submerged in the liquid.

6. Place a drop-lid or any lightweight lid on top, to anchor the *kabocha* pieces.

7. Bring to the boil, turn down to a simmer and cook for a further 10–15 minutes.

Measurements	Ingredients
800 g	*Kabocha* squash
Stock	
400 ml	Water
4 tbsp	Caster sugar
200 ml	*Sake*
2 tbsp	Japanese light soy sauce
Garnish	
½ tsp	Shredded *yuzu* rind (use tangerine if *yuzu* is unavailable)

8. When the liquid has reduced by two-thirds, add the light soy sauce.

9. Cook for another minute and coat the *kabocha* pieces with the reduced liquid, taking care not to burn them.

10. Serve warm, garnished with shredded *yuzu* (or tangerine) rind.

Quality Points

- *Kabocha* pieces should have a chestnut-like texture when cooked.
- They should be well coated with the stock and taste slightly sweet with a soy sauce overtone.

Chef's Tip

- Add the soy sauce at the end, and not any earlier, so that the dish will not taste salty. (See the key points on simmering on p. 25)

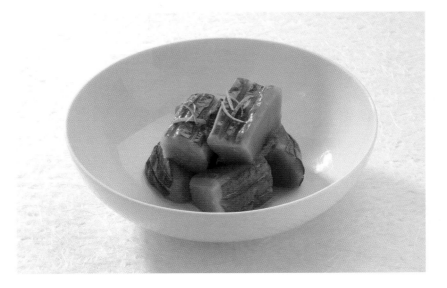

Sliced Daikon Radish Salad with Sanbai-zu Japanese Dressing 大根の三杯酢

Method

1. Rub the thinly sliced *daikon* radish (mooli) with the salt and leave for 10 minutes.

2. Rinse off the salt and squeeze hard to remove excess water.

3. Mix the lemon rind with the *daikon* slices.

4. Coat in the *sanbai-zu* dressing and arrange neatly on a serving dish. Garnish with the shredded *shiso* leaves and toasted sesame seeds.

Quality Points

• The *daikon* radish should be smooth and taste slightly lemony.

Chef's Tip

• Remove the pith, a source of bitterness, from the lemon rind. This salad goes well with a *teriyaki* dish.

Measurements	Ingredients
200 g	*Daikon* radish (mooli), peeled and sliced thinly using a mandolin
1 tbsp	Salt
1	Lemon, with the rind removed and cut into very fine strips (2–3 mm)
200 ml	*Sanbai-zu* dressing (see p. 42 for recipe)
Garnish	
4	*Shiso* (green perilla) leaves, finely shredded
1 tsp	Toasted white sesame seeds

Cold Poached Egg Starter 冷やし卵

This is a delicious starter for a hot summer's day.

Method

Measurements	Ingredients
1 litre	Water
1 tsp	Salt
2 tbsp	Vinegar
4	Large eggs
Condiment	
2 tbsp	Japanese soy sauce

1. Bring the water to the boil in a pan and then reduce the heat to a simmer.

2. Add the salt and vinegar to the water and mix well.

3. Carefully break the eggs one by one into the pan. Simmer for $2^{1/2}$–3 minutes.

4. Using a slotted spoon, transfer the eggs into a bowl of iced water.

5. Tidy up the eggs by trimming the white, if necessary. Refrigerate to chill.

6. To serve, place each egg in an ice-cold individual glass bowl with $^{1/2}$ tsp of soy sauce.

Japanese Rolled Omelette 厚焼き卵

This recipe will make 2 omelettes.

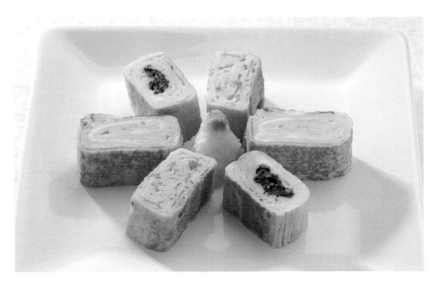

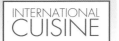

If possible, use a square Japanese omelette pan (see p. 23) for this omelette.

Method

1. Combine the eggs, sugar, *sake* and soy sauce in a mixing bowl. Beat until the sugar dissolves. Strain the liquid.

2. Heat a traditional square frying pan or a non-stick medium-sized frying pan and cover the base with a little vegetable oil.

3. Pour in enough of the egg mixture to cover the pan's base, tilting the pan to spread it evenly. Break any large air bubbles. When the mixture is almost set, run chopsticks or a spatula around edge of the pan to loosen the omelette.

4. Starting from the furthest side of the pan, fold over the omelette three times, moving it towards the near side of the pan. Gently push the folded omelette to the front of the pan.

Measurements	Ingredients
6	Eggs
2 tbsp	Caster sugar
2 tbsp	*Sake*
1 tbsp	Japanese light soy sauce
2 tbsp	Vegetable oil
Garnish	
2 tbsp	*Daikon* radish (mooli), finely grated
Condiment	
1 tsp	Japanese soy sauce

5. Lightly oil the pan again and repeat the procedure (keeping the already cooked omelette where it is in the pan), lifting the cooked omelette so that the egg mixture runs underneath it as well. When nearly cooked, fold the 'new' omelette over the first one, pushing this to the centre to form the core. Repeat this whole process a few times until the omelette is approximately 3 cm thick.

6. Tip the omelette on to a plate. Allow to cool. Cut into 2–3 cm slices and serve at room temperature with grated *daikon* radish and a dash of Japanese soy sauce.

Quality Points

- The omelette should be soft and moist inside when sliced.

Chef's Tip

- Sliced omelette is often used as a sushi topping or as a filling for thick sushi rolls when cut lengthways into long, thin strips. It is also served as part of a bento box lunch.

Variations

- **Spinach omelettes:** place blanched spinach in the centre and roll the omelette around it.

- **Spring onion omelettes:** add 2 tbsp of finely chopped spring onions to the egg solution and make the omelette as above.

Savoury Custard Cup 茶碗蒸し

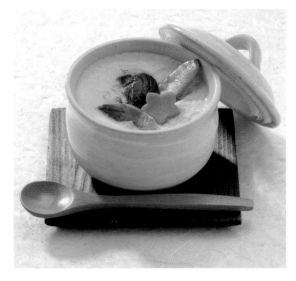

Measurements	Ingredients
Savoury custard	
400 ml	*Dashi* stock
1 tsp	Japanese light soy sauce
½ tsp	Salt
1 tsp	*Mirin*
2	Eggs
Fillings	
4	Small dried shiitake mushrooms
120 g	Chicken breast
1 tsp	Light soy sauce
120 g	White firm fish fillets (e.g. cod, pollock, haddock, coley)
½ tsp	Salt
4 slices	*Kamaboko* fish cakes
4	Fresh prawns
8	Gingko nuts
Garnish	
8	*Mitsuba* leaves or blanched flat parsley leaves

Preparation

- Prepare the following fillings and divide each equally into four portions.

- Reconstitute the dried mushrooms by soaking them in tepid water until soft, then remove the stalks.

- Cut the chicken into 2 cm pieces and sprinkle with the light soy sauce. Marinate for 5 minutes.

- Skin the fish fillets and cut into 3 cm pieces. Sprinkle with salt.

- Cut the *kamaboko* slices in half.

- Shell the prawns, leaving the tails on for decoration, then de-vein.

- Shell the gingko nuts and boil them in hot water for 5 minutes. Remove the thin skin and leave them to cool.

Method

1. Combine the *dashi* stock, soy sauce, salt and *mirin* together and mix well. Beat the eggs lightly, add the stock mixture, mix well and then strain.

2. Arrange the fillings in four individual cups and gently ladle the custard mixture over them.

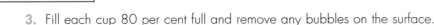

3. Fill each cup 80 per cent full and remove any bubbles on the surface.

4. Cover each cup with a lid or foil, place them on an oven tray and cook them in bains-marie (water bath) at a very low temperature (180C°) for 15–20 minutes, until the custard is just set.

5. Garnish with *mitsuba* leaves just before serving.

6. Serve hot in the individual lidded cups with a small spoon on the side.

Quality Points

• The custard should be just set – soft and still wobbly.

Chef's Tip

• The guideline for the egg-to-stock ratio is 1 part egg mixture to 3–4 parts stock. The *dashi* stock can be substituted with chicken stock for a richer taste. Light soy sauce is used so as not to colour the custard.

Soft Japanese Rolled Omelette だし巻き卵

This is a softer and fluffier version of the Japanese rolled omelette described on p. 124. This recipe makes two omelettes.

If possible, use a square Japanese omelette pan (see p. 23).

Method

1. Combine the eggs, *dashi* stock, sugar, salt and soy sauce in a mixing bowl. Beat until the sugar dissolves. Strain.

2. Heat a square omelette pan or a non-stick medium-sized frying pan and cover the base with a little oil.

3. Pour in enough of the egg mixture to cover the base of pan, tilting it to spread the mixture evenly. Break any large air bubbles that form. When the egg is almost set, run chopsticks or a spatula around the edge of the pan to loosen the omelette.

4. Starting from the furthest side of the pan, fold the omelette over three times, then gently push the folded omelette to the near side.

Measurements	Ingredients
4	Eggs
50 ml	*Dashi* stock
2 tbsp	Caster sugar
¼ tsp	Salt
1 tbsp	Japanese light soy sauce
2 tbsp	Vegetable oil
Garnish	
2 tbsp	*Daikon* radish (mooli), finely grated
Condiment	
1 tsp	Japanese soy sauce

5. Lightly oil the pan again and repeat the procedure (keeping the already cooked omelette where it is in the pan), lifting the cooked omelette so that the egg mixture runs underneath it as well. When nearly cooked, fold the 'new' omelette over the first one, pushing this to the centre to form the core. Repeat this whole process a few times until the omelette is approximately 3 cm thick.

6. Tip the omelette on to a plate. Allow to cool. Cut into 2–3 cm slices and serve at room temperature with grated *daikon* radish and a dash of Japanese soy sauce.

Quality Points

* The omelette should be soft and fluffy.

Chef's Tip

* Finely chopped spring onions can be added for texture and colour.

Assorted Tempura 天ぷら

To make successful *tempura*, ensure that all the ingredients are ice cold, the batter lumpy, and only a few pieces fried at a time. Any vegetable with a firm texture can be used.

In order to make a successful batter, note that all ingredients must be kept in the fridge until just before mixing.

Method

1. Combine all the ingredients for the dipping sauce in a pan and gently bring to the boil. Put aside and leave to cool.

2. Shell and de-vein the prawns. Keep the tails on. Make a few incisions on the underside of the prawns to prevent curling while cooking.

3. Cut the squid lengthways into strips 4–5 cm wide and cut into 2 cm-wide slices. Score each piece a few times.

4. Wipe the mushroom caps. Wash the *shiso* leaves and dry thoroughly.

5. Slowly heat the oil to 160°C.

6. Beat the egg yolk lightly and mix with the ice-cold water.

7. Add half the flour to the above and mix lightly. Add the rest of the flour all at once. Combine the flour and egg-water in a few big strokes using chopsticks or a fork. The batter should be lumpy and the flour should just loosely cling to the egg-water, as over-mixing will result in oily and mushy *tempura*.

8. To prevent the oil splattering, dry all the ingredients thoroughly with kitchen paper before deep-frying.

9. Dip a few vegetable pieces (the green pepper, courgette and mushrooms) at a time into the batter, and fry for about 1½ minutes or until just crisp and golden. Drain the *tempura* and keep warm.

Measurements	Ingredients
12	Large prawns
300 g	Squid, cleaned and skinned
8	Shiitake mushrooms, stalks removed
8	*Shiso* (green perilla) leaves
1	Green pepper, seeded and cut into 2.5 cm strips
1	Courgette, cut into 1 cm rounds
1.5 l	Vegetable oil for deep-frying
Batter	
1	Egg yolk
200 ml	Ice-cold water
100 g	Plain flour, sifted
Dipping sauce	
200 ml	*Dashi* stock
3 tbsp	*Mirin*
3 tbsp	Japanese soy sauce
½ tsp	Grated ginger
Condiments	
4 tbsp	*Daikon* radish (mooli), grated

10. Repeat the process with the prawns and squid.

11. Lower the heat slightly, dip one side of the *shiso* leaves in flour and then in batter and deep-fry until crisp.

12. Arrange the *tempura* on a serving dish garnished with a small peak of grated *daikon* radish, with the dipping sauce in a separate bowl.

Quality Points

- Serve immediately when piping hot. *Tempura* should be light, not oily.

Chef's Tip

- Use any leftover *tempura* for *tempura* on rice (see recipe on p. 173).

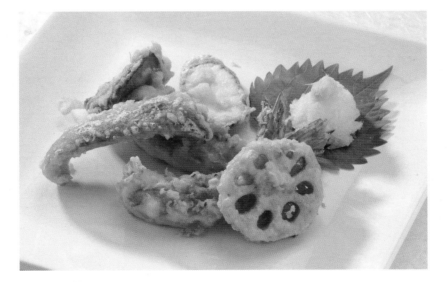

Braised Mackerel in Miso Sauce 鯖の味噌煮

Method

1. Sprinkle salt over the mackerel and leave in the fridge for 10 minutes.

2. Rinse off the salt and dry the mackerel with kitchen paper.

3. Pat each mackerel piece with potato starch.

4. Fry the fish in 150°C oil for 2–3 minutes or until the surface is slightly coloured. Drain on kitchen paper and put aside.

5. Add the *sake*, soy sauce, sugar and water into a shallow pan or skillet and bring to the boil over a medium heat. Add the ginger and simmer until it reaches boiling point.

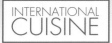
6. Dissolve the miso completely in a ladleful of the simmering liquid. Mix it into the liquid and add the *mirin*. Continue to simmer. Check the seasoning, adding salt if necessary.

7. Place the fried mackerel into the above and simmer until cooked. Add the potato starch mixed with water to thicken the sauce.

8. Serve the mackerel pieces on individual plates and ladle the sauce over them. Garnish with the spring onion and grated ginger.

Quality Points

- The mackerel should not be oily. The miso sauce is aromatic and slightly sweet with a hint of ginger.

Chef's Tip

- Do not overcook the miso sauce, as it will lose its flavour.

Measurements	Ingredients
	Salt
4	Mackerel darnes (steaks) weighing 120 g per portion
1 tbsp	Potato starch
	Vegetable oil for frying
Sauce	
3 tbsp	*Sake*
1 tbsp	Japanese soy sauce
3 tbsp	Caster sugar
300 ml	Water
5 cm	Ginger, shredded
1 tbsp	*Mirin*
3 tbsp	Miso
½ tsp	Potato starch mixed with 1 tbsp water
Garnish	
1	Spring onion, shredded
1 tbsp	Grated ginger

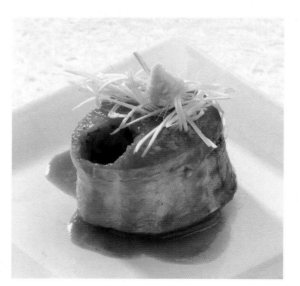

Cod Fillets En Papillote 鱈のホイル蒸し

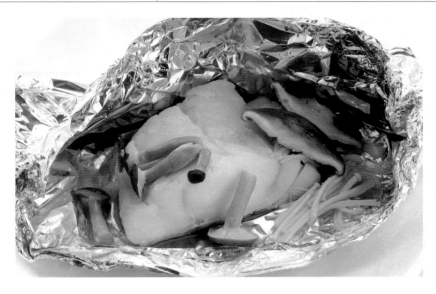

Preparation

- Remove the pin bones from the cod fillets and de-scale completely.

Method

1. Sprinkle salt on both sides of the cod fillets and leave for 10 minutes. (Salt cleanses the fish and makes it firmer.)

2. Rinse off the salt with water and dry thoroughly with kitchen paper.

3. Cut off 4 sheets of double-thickness aluminium foil 20 cm in length and place a fillet in the centre of each sheet.

4. Sprinkle the fish with the lemon juice, *sake* and soy sauce. Arrange the mushroom slices, spring onions, ginger strips and grated lime rind on top and leave for 15 minutes.

5. Loosely wrap the fish in the foil sheets, first folding it up in the middle and closing the two loose ends by rolling them up. Do not make the parcel too tight.

Measurements	Ingredients
2 tbsp	Salt
4	Cod fillets, each weighing 100–120 g with skin
2 tbsp	Lemon juice
4 tbsp	*Sake*
2 tbsp	Japanese soy sauce
4	Shiitake mushrooms, stalked and thinly sliced
4	Spring onions, thinly sliced diagonally
2 cm	Ginger, cut into julienne (strips)
1 tsp	Lime rind, finely grated
Garnish	
4 wedges	Lemon

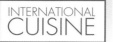

6. Place the wrapped fish in a steamer and heat for 10 minutes, or until cooked.

7. Transfer the parcels on to a serving plate garnished with lemon wedges. Break them open at the table and squeeze on the lemon juice. Serve immediately.

Quality Points

- Do not over-steam the fish to ensure that it will be moist and succulent when cooked.

Chef's Tip

- It is possible to substitute cod with any firm-textured white fish such as sea bream.

Salt-baked White Fish Fillets 塩釜焼き

Method

1. Combine the cooking salt and egg whites to form a mixture with the consistency of wet sand.

2. Place each fillet on a piece of silicon paper (or baking parchment) large enough to wrap it up. Sprinkle the fish with the salt, white pepper, sugar, *sake* and ginger juice.

3. Wrap up each fillet by folding in the two ends of the paper to the centre and then rolling together the two remaining ends tightly in order to trap the juice released during cooking.

4. Line an oven tray with foil and place the fish packages on it. Cover each package completely with the cooking salt/egg mix.

5. Bake the wrapped fish in the oven at 180°C for 20 minutes.

6. Place the fish packages on a large plate and serve.

7. Break open at the table.

Measurements	Ingredients
2 kg	Cooking salt
3–4	Egg whites
4	White fish fillets (bream, sole, halibut, turbot) weighing 100–120 g each
2	Spring onions, very finely sliced
Pinch	Salt
Pinch	Ground white pepper
Pinch	Caster sugar
1 tbsp	*Sake*
1 tsp	Ginger juice

Quality Points

- The fish should be succulent when cooked, and should have a delicate flavour of ginger and *sake*.

Chef's Tip

- Take care not to overcook, as salt retains heat when the fish is taken out of the oven. Fish fillets can be substituted with seafood if desired.

Salt-grilled Fish 魚の塩焼き

This basic technique can be applied to most fish with firm flesh.

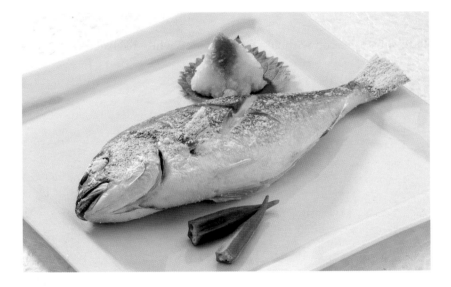

Method

1. Sprinkle the salt evenly over the whole fish. Put aside for 10 minutes until they start to sweat.

2. Wash the peppers, remove the stalks, de-seed and cut lengthways in half. Skewer crosswise on cocktail sticks.

3. Rinse the salt from the fish and pat dry with kitchen towels. Sprinkle a pinch of salt on each side of each fish again.

4. Pre-heat the grill to a high temperature and adjust the shelf to the optimum distance from the heat.

5. Place the fish on a wire rack over a baking tray and grill the side to be presented to the diner first, for about 5–6 minutes until 70 per cent cooked. (NB: a grilled whole fish is served to the diner with its head facing to the left.)

Measurements	Ingredients
4	Whole fish (e.g. sea bream, snapper or mackerel) with heads attached, each weighing 400–500 g, gutted and scaled
2 tbsp	Sea salt
Garnish	
4	Small bell chilli peppers or small yellow peppers
½ tsp	Vegetable oil
4 tbsp	Freshly grated *daikon* radish (mooli) divided into 4 portions
½ tsp	Japanese soy sauce

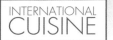
6. At the same time, grill the skewered peppers, brushing with vegetable oil and turning over once. This will take about 2 minutes.

7. When the fish become firm to the touch, are sweating and slightly coloured, turn them over and grill the other side until the skin is crisp and golden brown.

8. Arrange the fish on individual serving plates, garnished with grated *daikon* radish formed into a pyramid, and decorate the top with a drop of soy sauce. Remove the cocktail sticks from the peppers and place 2 halves with each whole fish.

Quality Points

- For good grilled fish, take care not to overcook, but ensure that the skin is crisp.

Chef's Tip

- Maintain the grill at a high heat, and adjust the position of the rack in order to achieve the heat level required. If bell peppers or small yellow peppers are unavailable, use blanched okra instead.

Simmered Flat Fish 鰈の煮付け

Method

1. De-scale, and gut the fish, rinse off the scales and blood. Cut into 10 cm *tronçons* (steaks). Score the skin diagonally twice on each piece.

2. Combine the water, sake, caster sugar, *mirin* and 2 tbsp of the soy sauce in a pan and bring to the boil. Slide in the fish and bring to the boil over a medium heat. Skim the stock, place a drop-lid on top of the fish and simmer for 12–13 minutes or until the liquid is reduced to one-third.

3. Add the remaining 1 tbsp of soy sauce and bring to the boil again. Take the pan off the heat.

4. Arrange the fish on a plate and pour over one or two tablespoonsful of the sauce. Garnish with ginger strips and blanched French beans.

Measurements	Ingredients
8	10 cm *tronçons* (steaks) of flat fish (plaice, dab etc.)
Simmering liquid	
200 ml	Water
4 tbsp	*Sake*
2 tbsp	Caster sugar
2 tbsp	*Mirin*
3 tbsp	Japanese soy sauce
Garnish	
2 cm	Ginger, cut into fine julienne (strips) and soaked in cold water
4–5	French beans (blanched) cut into 5 cm lengths

Chef's Tip

- This dish tastes better if cooked in advance, chilled and reheated before serving.

Sesame-flavoured Deep-fried Cod with Shredded Cabbage
鱈の胡麻フライと刻みキャベツ

Method

1. Cut the cod into 10 cm slices. Salt it on both sides and leave until it sweats. Rinse and dry thoroughly with kitchen paper.

2. Prepare three trays: the first containing the beaten egg, the second the potato starch seasoned with a pinch of ground white pepper and salt, and the third the mixture of the white untoasted sesame seeds and *panko* breadcrumbs.

3. Dip the cod slices in the potato starch first, then the egg mixture and finally in the sesame breadcrumbs. Ensure each slice is completely covered in crumbs.

4. Cover and put them in the fridge for 10–15 minutes so that the breadcrumbs do not come off while frying.

5. Wash the cabbage and shred it paper-thin using a mandolin. Soak in cold water until crisp and then drain. Dry with kitchen paper.

6. Heat the oil to 170°C. Slide in 2 or 3 fillets at a time. Deep-fry for about 5 minutes until golden brown, taking care not to burn the sesame seeds, and turning over the fillets once or twice. Skim the oil frequently.

7. Drain on absorbent paper.

8. On each serving plate, arrange a single fillet on a bed of cabbage, garnished with lemon wedges.

Measurements	Ingredients
4	Fillets of cod, weighing 100–120 g each
1 tbsp	Salt
	Vegetable oil, sufficient for deep-frying
Coating	
1	Egg, lightly beaten
4 tbsp	Potato starch
Pinch	Ground white pepper
Pinch	Salt
4 tbsp	Untoasted white sesame seeds
50 g	*Panko* breadcrumbs
Garnish	
8 leaves	Tender point cabbage, mandolin shredded
4	Lemon wedges

Quality Points

• The fried cod fillet should be light and crispy without being oily.

Chef's Tip

• Any fish of the cod family works well with this recipe.

Simmered Sardines with Ginger 鰯の生姜煮

Method

1. De-scale the sardines; neatly remove their heads and gut them. Rinse thoroughly in salted water.

2. Place the sardines flat, without overlapping, in a saucepan lined with silicon paper (or baking parchment).

3. Combine the ingredients for liquid 1 and pour over the sardines. Place a drop-lid on top and cook for 15 minutes. (This process reduces the strong flavour of the sardines.)

4. Drain, leaving the sardines in the pan.

5. Add the *sake* and water and bring to the boil. Reduce the heat, add the *mirin* and sugar, and cook for 10 minutes.

6. Add the soy sauce and ginger, and simmer until the liquid has almost evaporated. Chill.

7. Arrange the sardines on a plate and garnish with the shredded ginger. Serve at room temperature.

Measurements	Ingredients
1 kg	Small sardines of similar size
Liquid 1	
200 ml	Water
70 ml	Rice vinegar
Liquid 2	
200 ml	Water
2 tbsp	*Sake*
2 tbsp	*Mirin*
1½ tbsp	Sugar
4 tbsp	Japanese soy sauce
5 cm	Ginger, cut into fine juliennne (strips)
Garnish	
5cm	Ginger, shredded, soaked in cold water

Quality Points

• Ensure that the sardines do not break up while simmering so that they look neat and presentable on the plate. They should taste of sweet soy sauce with a hint of ginger.

Chef's Tip

• This makes a good starter.

Assorted Sashimi 刺身の盛り合わせ

Make sure that you use the freshest fish possible for this dish.

Method

1. Prepare the fillets for *sashimi* (see the *sashimi* filleting technique on p. 35).

2. *Sashimi*-slice the tuna to approximately 1 cm in thickness (see the *sashimi* slicing technique on p. 36).

3. Repeat the procedure with the sea bream.

4. *Sashimi*-slice the turbot.

5. Drain the shredded *daikon* radish and dry.

6. Heap the shredded radish on a serving plate. Place *shiso* leaves on top.

7. Arrange the tuna slices diagonally on the *shiso* leaves, placing the sea bream and turbot slices in the foreground. Garnish with a dollop of *wasabi* paste.

8. Serve cold with individual plates of soy sauce.

Measurements	Ingredients
200 g	Tuna fillet (a rectangular block 2.5 cm long and 5–6 cm wide)
200 g	Sea bream *sashimi* fillet
200 g	Turbot *sashimi* fillet
Garnish	
50 g	Very finely shredded *daikon* radish (mooli), soaked in cold water for 30 minutes
	Shiso (green perilla) leaves
Condiments	
1 tbsp	*Wasabi* paste
	Japanese soy sauce

Chef's Tip

• Keep the fillets in the fridge at the optimum 0–2°C until you start. Once out of the fridge, minimise handling.

Vinegared Mackerel Sashimi 鯖

Oily fish are offered vinegared when made into *sashimi*.

Method

1. Gut the mackerel and fillet it, using the three-pieces filleting technique (see p. 35).

2. Smother both sides of the two fillets with salt. Cover with cling film and leave in a fridge for 6 hours. Salt heavily for a successful result.

3. After 6 hours, the fish should have turned hard. Rinse off the salt in cold water and dry the fish thoroughly.

4. Wipe the surface dust off the *konbu* with a damp cloth.

5. Take a container large enough for the two fillets and line the bottom with sheets of *konbu*. Place

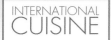

the fillets on top and cover with another layer of *konbu*.

6. Cover the fish completely with the *sanbai-zu* vinegar dressing. Leave for 2–3 hours.

7. After 2–3 hours, the flesh will have turned pale. Remove the pin bones and peel off the skin.

8. On each serving plate, arrange 2–3 tablespoonsful of shredded *daikon* radish, formed into a peak (slightly to one side, so there is room to sit the *sashimi* slices next to it), and a *shiso* leaf.

9. Dry the fillets thoroughly with kitchen paper, slice into 6 mm thicknesses, applying the *sashimi* slicing technique (see p. 36).

10. Serve about 6 slices per portion, next to the radish peak, placing a small knob of *wasabi* paste by the *sashimi*. Serve with a small plate of soy sauce.

Chef's Tip

- Be sure to use the freshest mackerel you can get. *Sashimi*-quality fish should be odourless.

Measurements	Ingredients
1	Very fresh whole mackerel weighing 400–500 g
3 tbsp	Salt
50 g	Dried *konbu* seaweed
200 ml	*Sanbai-zu* vinegar dressing (see the recipe on p. 42)
Garnish	
5 cm	*Daikon* radish (mooli), shredded and soaked in cold water for 30 minutes, then dried
4	*Shiso* (green perilla) leaves
Condiments	
1 tbsp	*Wasabi* powder mixed with a little water to form a stiff paste
	Japanese soy sauce

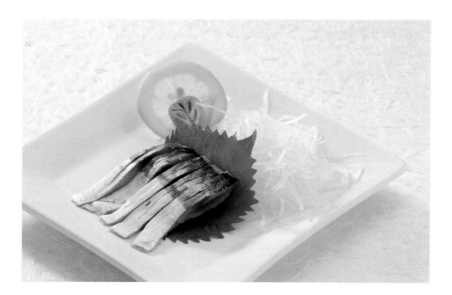

Teriyaki Salmon 鮭の照り焼き

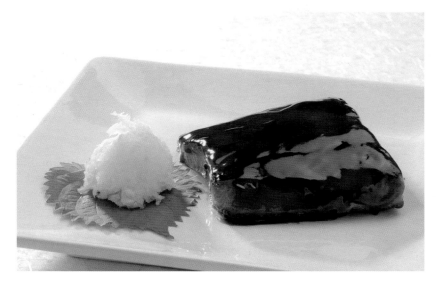

Method

1. Pre-heat the oven to 180°C.

2. Sprinkle the salt all over the salmon. Put aside until it starts to sweat.

3. Combine all the ingredients for the sauce, except the potato starch, in a pan and heat until the sugar is completely dissolved. Reduce the sauce by simmering for 2 minutes, and gradually add the diluted potato starch to thicken slightly. Cook for a further 1–2 minutes to remove any starchy taste.

4. Pre-heat the grill, and oil the grill rack to prevent the fish sticking to it.

5. Rinse the salmon with water to remove any salt from the surface. Pat dry with kitchen paper.

6. Place the fish in the grill and cook flesh side up until the surface is slightly coloured.

7. Remove the fish from the grill and transfer to an oiled oven tray.

Measurements	Ingredients
4	Salmon fillets, pin bones removed, weighing 120–150 g each
2 tbsp	Salt
Sauce	
2 tbsp	Japanese soy sauce
1 tbsp	*Mirin*
1 tbsp	Caster sugar
2 tbsp	Water
1 tsp	Potato starch diluted with 1 tbsp of water
Garnish	
2 tbsp	*Daikon* radish (mooli), freshly grated

8. Brush the sauce over the fish and dry the surface in the pre-heated oven, being careful not to burn the sauce.

9. Repeat step 8 until the fish is cooked and looks glossy.

10. Serve the fish fillets on individual plates garnished with freshly grated *daikon* radish on the side.

Quality Points

- The fish should be glossy and evenly coloured. It should be cooked through, but remain moist and succulent.

Steamed White Fish and Tofu with Ponzu Sauce ちり蒸し

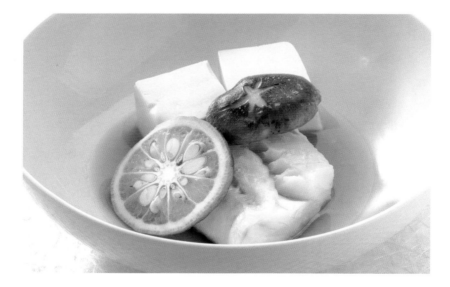

Method

1. Wipe the *konbu* squares with a damp cloth to remove any dust, and put aside.

2. Cut the tofu into 4 cm cubes.

3. Sprinkle salt evenly over the tofu squares, fish fillets and mushrooms, and leave for about 10 minutes.

4. Divide the above ingredients into four portions.

5. Place one *konbu* square in each serving bowl. Place one portion of the tofu, fish and shiitake mixture on top of the *konbu* in each bowl. Garnish with a slice of *yuzu* (or lemon or lime).

6. Cover and cook in a steamer for 11–12 minutes.

7. When cooked, spoon the *ponzu* sauce over the top. Serve hot.

Quality Points

- Tofu, fish and mushrooms should not be overcooked.

Measurements	Ingredients
4	5 cm squares dried *konbu*
250 g	Tofu (firm cotton type)
	Salt
4	Firm white fish fillet (cod, haddock, sea bream or sea bass), scaled, skinned, each weighing 100–120 g
4	Shiitake mushrooms, stems removed
180 ml	*Ponzu* sauce (see recipe on p. 43)
Garnish	
4 slices	Citrus fruits (*yuzu*, lemon or lime)

Braised Japanese Vegetables with Chicken
筑前煮

Preparation

* Sprinkle salt over the *konnyaku* and soften by pounding it a few times with a rolling pin. Wash off the salt and rinse under warm water. Cut in half lengthways and then slice into 1 cm thicknesses and dry-toast in a pan until the excess moisture evaporates.

Method

1. Heat the oil in a medium-sized saucepan over a high heat until very hot and stir-fry the chicken first, then the *konnyaku* pieces, mushrooms, carrots, bamboo shoots and burdock, in that order.

2. Sir-fry for about 3 minutes until all the ingredients are well coated with oil and partially cooked.

3. Pour in the *dashi* stock so that it barely covers the chicken and vegetables.

4. Bring to the boil over a high heat, add the sugar and cook for 2–3 minutes, then add the soy sauce.

5. Put a drop-lid or a small light plate wrapped with foil, on top and simmer until the liquid is reduced by one-third.

6. Remove from the heat. Mix in the par-boiled peas for colour just before serving.

7. Serve either hot or at room temperature in individual dishes, making sure the various ingredients are arranged attractively on each dish.

Measurements	Ingredients
2 tbsp	Vegetable oil
200 g	Boned chicken thighs, cut into 2.5 cm pieces
1 sheet	*Konnyaku*
6	Dried shiitake mushrooms, reconstituted
100 g	Carrots, roll-cut (see p. 28) into 2 cm pieces
50 g	Bamboo shoots, cut into 2 cm chunks
1	Burdock (optional), scrubbed and cut into 2 cm diagonal slices
200 ml	*Dashi* stock
2 tbsp	Caster sugar
4 tbsp	Japanese soy sauce
50 g	Frozen peas, par-boiled

Quality Points

- Chicken and vegetables should be al dente. The dish should not be oily.

Chef's Tip

- This dish allows diners to enjoy a variety of textures and is often part of a bento box meal.

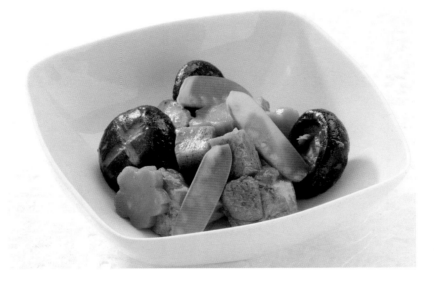

Deep-fried Breadcrumbed Chicken 鶏カツ

This is the chicken version of the famous *tonkatsu*.

Preparation

- Wash and shred the cabbage paper-thin using a mandolin or slicer. Soak in cold water for 15 minutes to make it crisp, and then drain.
- Prepare three trays, each with one of the three coating ingredients: first, the flour seasoned with the ground pepper and salt; second, the lightly beaten eggs; and, third, the *panko* breadcrumbs. Line them up.

Method

1. Place the chicken breasts on a flat surface and wrap each one in cling film. Then hit each piece gently with a rolling pin until all the breasts are flattened to uniform thickness. Unwrap.

2. Line up the three trays of coating ingredients. Lift a chicken breast piece with a cocktail stick and dredge the chicken in the flour. Shake off any excess. Next dip it into the beaten egg and then into the breadcrumbs, making sure the chicken is entirely coated in breadcrumbs. Repeat for each chicken breast.

3. Cover and refrigerate the chicken for 30 minutes.

4. Heat the oil in a heavy-bottomed cast-iron pot or deep-fryer to 170–175°C. Slide in 2 chicken pieces and deep-fry them until golden for about 5 minutes. Turn over the chicken once during frying to ensure an even-coloured finish, skimming the oil frequently to keep it clean.

5. Drain the chicken on kitchen paper. Keep hot.

6. Slice the chicken crosswise in 2 cm thicknesses, if serving in the Japanese style. Otherwise, serve each breast whole.

7. Arrange a half-plate full of shredded cabbage, formed into a mound on each plate.

8. Place a chicken breast against the cabbage and garnish with a lemon wedge.

9. Serve very hot.

Measurements	Ingredients
4	Chicken breasts, 100–120 g each
2 litres	Vegetable oil for deep-frying
Coating	
4 tbsp	Plain flour
Pinch	Ground white pepper
Pinch	Salt
2	Eggs, lightly beaten
100 g	*Panko* breadcrumbs
Garnish	
1	Tenderpoint cabbage
1	Lemon, cut into 4 wedges

Quality Points

- The chicken breasts should be light, not oily, and moist and succulent on the inside.

Deep-fried Chicken Goujons 鶏肉の胡麻揚げ

Method

1. Slice the chicken breast into goujons (strips).

2. Add the salt, pepper, sugar, a pinch of the potato starch and the *sake* to the chicken strips, mix thoroughly and marinate for 30 minutes.

3. Prepare three trays: the first containing potato starch, the second the beaten egg, the third a mixture of the untoasted white sesame seeds and the *panko* breadcrumbs.

4. Dip the chicken strips in the potato starch first, then the egg and finally the sesame breadcrumbs. Make sure the strips are well coated with the crumbs.

5. Repeat with all the chicken strips.

6. Put them in the fridge for 10–15 minutes.

7. Heat the oil in a heavy-bottomed cast-iron pot or deep-fryer to 160–170°C. Slowly add the chicken a few pieces at a time and fry for 3–4 minutes until cooked and the sesame seeds are golden. Drain on kitchen paper. Repeat this procedure with the remaining chicken.

8. Serve hot, garnishing each plate with a lemon wedge and *ponzu* sauce on the side.

Measurements	Ingredients
400 g	Chicken breast
2 litres	Vegetable oil for deep-frying
Marinade	
1 tsp	Salt
Dash	Ground white pepper
½ tsp	Caster sugar
Pinch	Potato starch
1 tsp	*Sake*
Coating	
1	Egg, beaten
3–4 tbsp	Potato starch
5 tbsp	Untoasted white sesame seeds
100 g	*Panko* breadcrumbs
Condiments	
	Ponzu sauce (see recipe on p. 43)
Garnish	
1	Lemon, cut into 4 wedges

Quality Points

- The chicken should be succulent inside and crisp and light on the outside, not oily. The sesame seeds should not be burnt.

Chef's Tip

- Fry in advance and freeze for reheating in the oven just before serving.

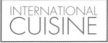
Deep-fried Marinated Chicken (Chicken Tatsuta-age) 竜田揚げ

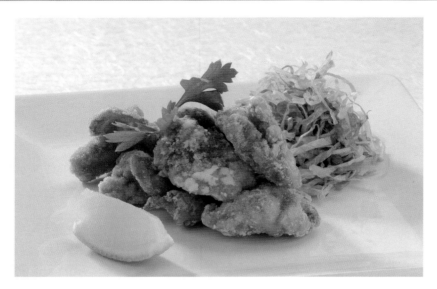

Preparation

- Peel and grate the ginger very finely and squeeze out the juice.

- Combine the ingredients for the marinade and mix well.

- Cut the chicken into 5 cm pieces with the skin attached. Mix the chicken pieces thoroughly with the marinade, using both hands. Leave to stand for 2–3 hours.

Method

1. Drain the chicken of the marinade and dust the individual pieces lightly with potato starch. Let the coated pieces rest in the fridge for 20 minutes.

2. Heat the oil in a deep-fryer to a medium temperature (160–170°C).

3. Slide the chicken into the hot oil, a few pieces at a time. Turn and separate the individual

Measurements	Ingredients
400 g	Boned chicken with skin
3 tbsp	Potato starch
2 litres	Vegetable oil for deep-frying
Marinade	
3 tbsp	*Sake*
1 tbsp	Japanese soy sauce
½ tbsp	Fresh ginger juice
1 tbsp	Spring onion, finely chopped
Garnish	
1	Lemon, cut into 4 wedges
1 sprig	Parsley
4 leaves	Lettuce, finely shredded

pieces as they fry until they are cooked and golden in colour. Skim the oil frequently. Drain the chicken on kitchen paper and keep hot.

4. To serve, place 6 to 8 pieces of chicken on a bed of shredded lettuce on each individual plate. Garnish each with a lemon wedge and a sprig of parsley.

Quality Points

- The chicken should be light and crisp, not oily, with an aroma of ginger and soy sauce.

Chef's Tip

- This recipe works well with chicken wings or drum sticks for serving in a buffet. Make sure the oil is not too hot otherwise the chicken will burn before it is cooked.

Grilled Marinated Duck 鴨の山椒焼き

Method

1. Combine the marinade ingredients and heat gently over a low heat to dissolve the sugar and burn off the alcohol in the *sake*. Leave to cool.

2. Trim any excess fat from the duck breast and tidy up the shape.

3. Score the duck skin. Rub in the salt, sugar and *sansho* pepper well. Leave aside for 3–4 hours.

4. Pour the boiling water over the duck skin and dry with kitchen paper.

5. Place the duck in the marinade and leave overnight. Retain the marinade.

6. Heat the vegetable oil in a non-stick frying pan and cook the duck, skin side only, until golden brown and crispy. Remove from the pan and drain off fat completely.

7. Return the duck to a clean frying pan and cook the flesh side slowly until it is cooked and brown outside.

Measurements	Ingredients
400 g	Duck breast, skin on
½ tsp	Salt
¼ tsp	Caster sugar
½ tsp	Ground *sansho* pepper
1 tbsp	Vegetable oil
	Boiling water
Marinade	
75 ml	Japanese soy sauce
4 tbsp	Caster sugar
100 ml	*Sake*
Garnish	
	Rocket leaves or watercress (enough to add decorative garnish)

8. Meanwhile, bring the retained marinade to the boil and simmer until slightly thickened. Strain through muslin. Check the seasoning and adjust if necessary. Keep warm.

9. Slice the duck and arrange neatly on serving plates garnished with rocket leaves. Spoon the marinade over. Serve hot.

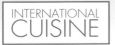
Method

1. Thread the chicken and vegetables on to 20 bamboo skewers, leaving space between the pieces.

2. Combine the sauce ingredients in a small pan and bring to the boil. Simmer the liquid so that the sauce thickens and is reduced by half.

3. Cook the skewers in small batches on a grill or barbecue, turning and basting with the sauce using a brush until the meat and vegetables are browned all over and cooked through.

4. Arrange 2–3 skewers of the *yakitori* on a plate with the condiments so that the peppers can be sprinkled according to individual taste.

5. Serve hot.

The following recipe offers a variation.

Measurements	Ingredients
500 g	Chicken thighs or breast, cut into 2.5 cm square pieces
100 g	Shiitake mushrooms, stalks removed and cut in half
6	Spring onions, cut into 2.5 cm lengths
Sauce	
5 tbsp	Japanese soy sauce
4 tbsp	Sake
2½ tbsp	Mirin
2 tbsp	Caster sugar
Condiments	
	Ground *sansho* pepper
	Shichimi pepper

Minced Chicken Balls (Tsukune) つくね

Method

1. Food-process the chicken to a smooth and sticky paste.

2. Add the bicarbonate of soda, potato starch, *sake*, salt and spring onion, and mix well. Leave to marinate for 1 hour.

3. Make the mixture into balls (2 cm in diameter) and poach them in simmering water until cooked. Leave the meatballs to cool.

4. Thread the cooked meatballs on to bamboo skewers. Grill or barbecue, continuing to baste with the *yakitori* sauce until browned and heated through.

5. Arrange them and serve as for *yakitori*, above.

Measurements	Ingredients
200 g	Chicken breast
Pinch	Bicarbonate of soda
1 tsp	Potato starch
1 tbsp	Sake
Pinch	Salt
2 tbsp	Spring onion, finely chopped
1 litre	Water
	Yakitori sauce (see recipe above)

Quality Points

- Ensure all ingredients are cooked through and well basted.

Steamed Chicken with Ginger-flavoured Soy Sauce 蒸し鶏

Method

1. Prick the chicken skin all over with a fork.

2. Cut the garlic clove in half and use it to rub the chicken surface. Marinade the chicken legs in the *sake* for 10–15 minutes.

3. Sprinkle the salt and sugar over the chicken and cook in a steamer for 15 minutes or until the chicken is just cooked. (The cooking time depends on the thickness of the meat.)

4. Cool the chicken in its own juices. During the cooling, be sure to cover the chicken to prevent the surface drying out.

5. Cut the chicken into 2 cm slices. Arrange these neatly on a bed of lettuce and serve with the ginger-flavoured soy sauce on the side.

Measurements	Ingredients
4	Boned chicken legs with skin (about 120 g each)
1 clove	Garlic
4 tbsp	*Sake* (to marinade)
Pinch	Salt
1 tsp	Caster sugar
Accompanying sauce	
4 tbsp	Ginger-flavoured soy sauce (see p. 45 for recipe)
Garnish	
4	Cos lettuce leaves, shredded

Quality Points

- The chicken should be moist and succulent.

Chef's Tip

- This makes a nice starter in hot weather. The leftover chicken can be used in salads.

Steamed Stuffed Shiitake Mushrooms
蒸し椎茸

Preparation

- Remove the skin and sinew from the chicken.

- Food-process the chicken to make a smooth mince.

- Combine the mince with the marinade ingredients and mix until slightly sticky. Add the beaten egg.

- Leave in the fridge for 2–3 hours or overnight.

Method

1. Remove the stalks from the shiitake mushrooms.

2. Stuff the mushroom cups with the mince, brush with sesame oil and decorate with sesame seeds.

3. Steam the stuffed mushrooms in a steamer for 10 minutes.

4. Serve them immediately on a bed of lettuce, with *ponzu* sauce on the side.

Quality Points

- The mince should look firm when cooked, providing a contrast in texture with the soft mushrooms.

Chef's Tip

- Meatballs or chicken burgers can be made with any leftover mince.

Measurements	Ingredients
100 g	Chicken leg meat, boned
1	Egg white, beaten
16	Shiitake mushrooms
Marinade	
½ tsp	Potato starch
1 tsp	Salt
1 tsp	Caster sugar
½ tsp	*Sake*
Pinch	Bicarbonate of soda
1 tsp	Japanese soy sauce
Glaze	
1 tsp	Sesame oil
Garnish	
½ tsp	Toasted white sesame seeds
2	Cos lettuce leaves
Condiment	
	Ponzu sauce (see recipe on p. 43)

Stuffed Lotus Roots with Minced Chicken
蓮根のはさみ揚げ

Preparation

- Remove any sinew from the chicken and cut the meat into small chunks. Food-process the chicken to make a fine mince.

- Combine the mince with the marinade ingredients and mix until slightly sticky. Then add the beaten egg white.

- Leave in the fridge for 2–3 hours or overnight.

Method

1. Wash and peel the lotus root.

2. Cut the root into 5 mm slices and leave in water to prevent discolouration.

3. Dry the slices and sandwich the prepared mince between two slices as if making an Oreo cookie, 1.5–2 cm thick. Take care the filling does not ooze out of the lotus root holes or at the edges.

4. Dust the stuffed lotus slices lightly with potato starch and shallow fry for 2–3 minutes until cooked and golden.

5. Arrange them on a bed of shredded lettuce and garnish with lemon wedges on a plate. Serve hot.

Quality Points

- The lotus root should be light and crunchy while the filling should be cooked without being dry.

Chef's Tip

- This is a dish that allows diners to enjoy textural contrast – the crunchiness of lotus root and the softness of the mince.

Measurements	Ingredients
100 g	Chicken leg meat
20 cm	Lotus root
1	Egg white, beaten
2 tbsp	Potato starch
Marinade	
¼ tsp	Potato starch
1 tsp	Salt
1 tsp	Sugar
½ tsp	*Sake*
Pinch	Bicarbonate of soda
1 tsp	Japanese soy sauce
Dash	Sesame oil
	Vegetable oil for frying
Garnish	
1	Lemon, cut into 4 wedges
4 leaves	Cos lettuce, finely shredded

Beef Tataki (Seared Beef) 牛肉のタタキ

This is beef sashimi.

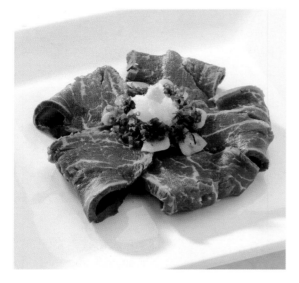

Measurements	Ingredients
300 g	Beef sirloin, fillet, cut to a rectangular-shaped block
½ tsp	Salt
Pinch	Ground white pepper
½ tbsp	Vegetable oil
1 tbsp	*Sake*
2 tbsp	Japanese soy sauce
1 tbsp	*Mirin*
Condiments	
1–2 cloves	Garlic, grated
6	Spring onions (green part only), very finely chopped
5 tbsp	Freshly grated *daikon* radish (mooli) mixed with grated, seeded red chilli
Garnish	
2	Spring onions, finely sliced
2–3 thin slices	Garlic
5 cm	Ginger, peeled and grated
1 tsp	Grated *daikon* radish (mooli)

Method

1. Rub the beef with the salt and ground white pepper.

2. Heat a frying pan over a low heat and pour in the oil, making sure the entire surface of the pan is coated.

3. Add the beef and sear quickly on all sides, making sure it is evenly browned.

4. Plunge the beef into ice-cold water to arrest cooking. Pat the beef dry.

5. Pour the *sake*, soy sauce and *mirin* into a pan, and bring to the boil once. Remove from the heat.

6. Put the beef back in the pan, coat it well with the sauce and cover tightly.

7. Leave the beef in the liquid and allow it to cool to room temperature.

8. Remove the beef from the liquid and pat it dry. Slice the beef paper-thin. Strain off the liquid and reserve.

9. Fold each slice of beef in half and arrange 'concentrically' on a serving plate.

10. Garnish each beef slice with the spring onion slices, garlic slices, grated ginger and grated *daikon*.

11. Just before serving, pour the reserved sauce over the beef. Serve with the condiments on the side.

Quality Points

- The beef should be tender and rare, cooked only on its outer surface. The sauce should be rich with a sweet overtone.

Chef's Tip

- Be sure to use good-quality beef and slice it paper-thin.

Braised Beef with Potatoes 肉じゃが

Method

1. Trim the fat from the beef and keep the fat. Cut beef into 5 cm squares

2. Bevel the edges of the potatoes and carrots (see p. 29).

3. Blanch the beef in hot water for 30 seconds, then refresh in cold water. Drain and put aside.

4. Blanch the onion slices in hot water for 30 seconds, then refresh in cold water. Drain and put aside.

5. Blanch the potatoes, carrots and *shira-taki* separately, refreshing in cold water afterwards. Drain and put aside.

6. Sauté the potatoes in the beef fat for 2–3 minutes and then discard the fat.

7. Add the *dashi* stock and water to the potatoes so that they are submerged in the liquid. Bring to the boil and simmer.

Measurements	Ingredients
200 g	Beef, topside thinly sliced (0.5 cm thickness)
800 g	Potatoes, cut into quarters
100 g	Carrots, round cut (see p. 28)
50 g	Onions, very thinly sliced
50 g	*Shira-taki* (see p. 67), cut into 5 cm lengths
150 ml	*Dashi* stock
150 ml	Water
3 tbsp	Caster sugar
2 tbsp	Japanese soy sauce
1 tbsp	*Mirin*
Garnish	
2 tbsp	Peas, blanched

8. When the potatoes start to change colour add the carrot and *shira-taki*, and continue to simmer for 2 minutes.

9. Add the sugar and onions and simmer for a further 3 minutes.

10. Add the soy sauce and *mirin*, and continue to cook for another minute. Return the beef to the pan.

11. Simmer until the potatoes are cooked and the stock is reduced to one-third. Adjust the seasoning and garnish with the peas.

12. Serve hot in individual bowls.

Quality Points

• The vegetables should not be overcooked, retaining their shape. They should be well seasoned.

Chef's Tip

• Chicken can be used instead of beef.

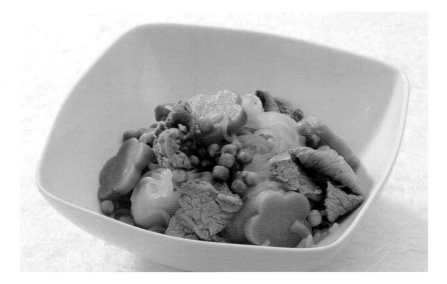

Braised Pork Belly in Miso 豚肉の味噌煮

Method

1. Trim the pork and cut it into 5 cm cubes. Blanch in boiling water for 5 minutes and drain.

2. Place the pork and shredded ginger in a clean pan. Cover with the *shochu*. If insufficient to immerse the pork, add water. Bring to the boil, cover with a drop-lid and simmer until the liquid is reduced by half. Skim all the time.

3. Dissolve the *miso* and sugar in a ladleful of the simmered liquid and mix in. Continue to simmer.

4. Sauté the onion slices in the vegetable oil until they are almost caramelised.

5. Combine the stir-fried onion with the pork and heat through. Check the reduced stock to see if it is slightly sweet. If it is still salty, add more sugar.

6. Arrange the pork on a serving plate and garnish with the diagonally sliced spring onion and grated ginger.

Measurements	Ingredients
500 g	Pork belly, trimmed and cut into 5 cm cubes
5 cm	Ginger, shredded
300 ml	Japanese *shochu* liquor or Chinese Shao Xing wine
5 tbsp	Caster sugar
60 g	*Akadashi miso*
100 g	Onion, very thinly sliced
3 tbsp	Vegetable oil
Garnish	
4	Spring onions, thinly sliced diagonally, soaked in cold water and drained
2 tsp	Ginger, grated

Quality Points

- The pork should be tender. The texture and flavour of onion and pork should contrast well with the miso and ginger.

Chef's Tip

- This dish tastes better when made in advance and reheated. Make sure it is not salty.

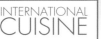
Deep-fried Breadcrumbed Pork Loin (Tonkatsu) とんかつ

Preparation

- Wash and shred the cabbage paper-thin using a mandolin or slicer. Soak the shredded cabbage in cold water for 15 minutes to make it crisp. Drain.

- Prepare three trays of the three different coatings: first the flour seasoned with the ground pepper and salt; second, the lightly beaten eggs; third, the panko breadcrumbs. Line them up.

Method

1. If tenderloin is used, slice it into 2 cm slices. If loin steaks are used, make a few incisions in the fat to prevent curling when deep-fried.

2. Line up the three trays of coatings. Lift a pork piece with a cocktail stick and dredge with the seasoned flour. Shake off any excess. Then dip the pork into the beaten egg and, finally, transfer to the last tray for coating entirely in breadcrumbs.

3. Cover and refrigerate the breadcrumbed pork for 30 minutes.

4. Heat the oil in a heavy-bottomed cast-iron pot or a deep fryer to 170–175°C. Slide in two steaks or four or five tenderloin slices, deep-fry for 5–7 minutes until golden. The pork should be turned over once or twice during frying to ensure an even-coloured finish. Skim the oil frequently to keep it clean.

5. Drain the deep-fried pork on absorbent kitchen paper. Keep warm.

6. If serving Japanese style, cut the pork crosswise into bite-sized slices, about 2 cm wide, or leave it uncut for European style.

7. Arrange a half-plate full of shredded cabbage in a mound and place the pork against it, with a spoonful of freshly prepared English mustard on the side. Add a lemon wedge to garnish. Either pour the *tonkatsu* sauce in a thin stream over the pork or place in a separate dish on the side.

8. Serve piping hot.

Measurements	Ingredients
4	Boned, 1.5 cm thick pork loin steaks, each weighing 120 g, or 400 g tenderloin, sliced into 2 cm rounds
2 litres	Vegetable oil for frying
Coatings	
4 tbsp	Plain flour
Pinch	Ground white pepper
Pich	Salt
2	Eggs, lightly beaten
100 g	*Panko* breadcrumbs
Garnish	
1	Tenderpoint cabbage
1	Lemon, cut into 4 wedges
Accompanying sauce	
1 tbsp	*Tonkatsu* sauce or Worcester sauce
Condiments	
4 tsp	Freshly prepared English mustard
4 tbsp	Japanese soy sauce

Quality Points

- The meat should be moist and succulent underneath its light and crispy crumb coating.

Chef's Tip

- Chicken can be used instead of pork. For a light and even-coloured finish, the fryer should contain oil 7–8 cm deep. Use any leftover *tonkatsu* for *katsu-don* (see the recipe on p. 170.)

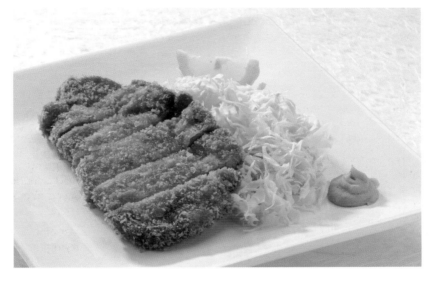

Pork and Choy-sum in Mustard-flavoured Miso Sauce 豚肉と小松菜の辛子味噌あえ

Method

1. Make the mustard-flavoured miso dressing according to the recipe on p. 44.

2. Blanch the *choy-sum* in slightly salted boiling water. Drain and cool in cold water to arrest cooking.

3. Squeeze out excess water and cut the *choy-sum* into 2 cm lengths. Coat with a small amount of soy sauce and squeeze out any remaining water.

4. Cut the pork into 3 cm-wide strips and swish them in the boiled water, making sure that the pan is off the heat. Cool the pork in the liquid so that it does not get tough.

5. When the pork has cooled, drain and dry completely with kitchen paper.

6. Combine the pork, *choy-sum* and spring onion, and mix well with the mustard-flavoured miso dressing.

7. Divide up into small individual bowls and serve at room temperature.

Quality Points

- The pork should be moist and tender and the vegetables al dente. All should be well coated with the dressing.

Chef's Tip

- Be sure to squeeze out any excess moisture from the *choy-sum* and pork to prevent the dish becoming watery.

Measurements	Ingredients
4 tbsp	Mustard-flavoured miso dressing (see p. 44 for the recipe)
100 g	*Choy-sum* Chinese greens, washed
1 tsp	Japanese soy sauce
200 g	Pork loin or shoulder, thinly sliced (5 mm thickness)
Garnish	
2	Spring onion, very thinly sliced

Pork Loin with Ginger-flavoured Soy Sauce
豚肉の生姜焼き

Method

1. Combine the marinade ingredients in a bowl and mix well.

2. Make incisions along the fat of the pork slices to prevent curling during cooking. Marinate for 20 minutes.

3. Heat the oil in a frying pan and sear the marinated pork slices on one side. Turn them over and add the soy sauce and *mirin*. Simmer until the pork is cooked, making sure it is well coated with the sauce.

4. Arrange the pork slices on individual plates and garnish with ginger strips.

Quality Points

- The pork should be succulent and well coated with the sauce.

Measurements	Ingredients
400 g	Boned long pork loin without rind, sliced to 1 cm thicknesses
2 tbsp	Vegetable oil
Marinade	
4 tbsp	Japanese soy sauce
2 tbsp	*Sake*
20 g	Ginger, finely grated
Sauce	
1½ tbsp	Japanese soy sauce
1½ tbsp	*Mirin*
Garnish	
2–3 slices	Ginger, shredded and soaked in water for 30 minutes

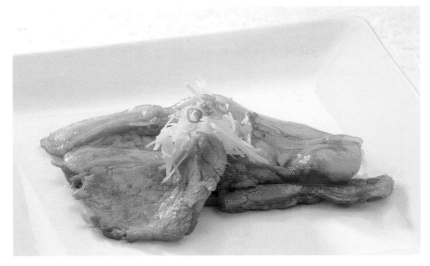

Shabu-shabu　しゃぶしゃぶ

This dish, cooked on the tabletop, offers diners an ideal opportunity for the appreciation of high-quality beef. You will need an earthenware pot or cast-iron skillet, and a tabletop burner.

Method

1. Cut the beef slices into 5 cm lengths and fold in half. Arrange the folded slices neatly on a large platter.

2. Arrange all the vegetables on another platter.

3. Place at the centre of the dining table the burner, the skillet, the beef and vegetable platters, and the two dipping sauces. Each diner is given two serving bowls into which to transfer individual portions of the two sauces.

4. Place the skillet on the burner and pour in hot water.

5. Allow the water to simmer to the boil and continue for 2–3 minutes.

6. To eat, each diner lifts a beef slice with chopsticks and swishes it in the simmering water a couple of times until the beef is cooked rare.

7. They then dip the beef in either of the two sauces before eating.

Measurements	Ingredients
600 g	High-quality well-marbled sirloin beef, cut into 1mm slices
100 g	Chinese leaves, with leaves and stalk separated and cut into uniform 1 cm x 2.5 cm strips
4	Spring onions, uniformly cut into 2.5 cm lengths
8	Shiitake mushrooms
250 g	Fresh tofu
200 g	Cooked fine *udon* noodles (see p. 62)
Sauces	
	Ponzu dipping sauce (see p. 43 for recipe)
	Ground sesame dipping sauce (see p. 43)

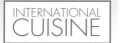

8. Every now and then vegetables and tofu are added to the stock in small quantities and eaten with the dipping sauces when cooked. Occasionally skim off the scum.

9. Repeat this process until all the beef slices and the rest of the ingredients, except the noodles, are eaten up.

10. Bring the stock to the boil. Drop in the *udon* noodles and let them soak up the broth. Eat to round off the meal.

Quality Points

• The beef slices should be eaten rare.

Simmered Spicy Pork Loin with Mustard Soy Sauce 煮豚

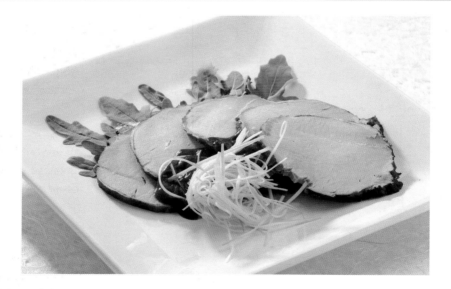

Method

1. Drop the tea bags in a pan containing sufficient water to cover the meat. Boil the water to brew the tea and then discard the bags.

2. Put the pork in the pan, ensuring that it is well immersed in the tea, and bring to the boil. Simmer for 20 minutes.

3. Take out the pork and drain. Discard the liquid.

4. Put the blanched pork in a clean pan and add the spices, soy sauce, *sake*, sugar, spring onion and ginger. Then pour on enough chicken stock to cover the meat.

5. Bring to the boil and simmer until the meat is cooked, skimming frequently.

6. Chill the meat in the liquid and store overnight in the fridge.

7. To make the accompanying sauce, completely dissolve the English mustard in the soy sauce. Add the water and mix well, then drop in a dash of sesame oil.

8. Remove the chilled pork from the fridge and drain off the stock. Retain the stock for making broth or to use as the base stock for egg noodle soup (*ramen*).

9. *To serve hot*: reheat the pork in the stock and slice into 2 cm thicknesses or as required. Arrange the slices neatly on a bed of rocket leaves and garnish with the shredded spring onions and the sauce.

10. *To serve cold*: slice and serve as cold cuts, European style, or use as a topping for soup noodles.

Quality Points

- The meat should be moist and succulent. It should be spicy with a sweet overtone.

Chef's Tips

- This is a very economical and versatile dish and it can be made well in advance.

Measurements	Ingredients
500 g	Rolled pork (loin, shoulder or neck)
2	Tea bags
	Water, enough to cover the meat
1	Star anise
1	Chinese brown cardamom seed
3 cm	*Cassia* bark or cinnamon
3	*Sichuan* peppercorns
100 ml	Japanese soy sauce
100 ml	*Sake*
3 tbsp	Caster sugar
1	Spring onion
3 cm	Ginger, thinly sliced
1–2 litres	Chicken stock
Sauce	
1 tbsp	Freshly prepared English mustard
3 tbsp	Japanese soy sauce
1 tbsp	Water
1–2 drops	Sesame oil
Garnish	
50 g	Rocket leaves
4	Spring onions (white part only), finely shredded, soaked in water for 10 minutes, drained and dried

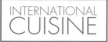
Stir-fried Beef with Ground Sansho Pepper
牛肉の有馬焼き

Method

1. Combine all the ingredients for the marinade and mix well. Place the sliced beef in the marinade, make sure it is well covered in it, and leave to stand for 30 minutes.

2. Heat half the oil in a wok and stir-fry the beef until almost done. Put aside and keep warm.

3. Heat the remainder of the oil in a clean wok and stir-fry the aubergine and pepper until cooked.

4. Add the beef to the vegetables and mix well. Add the soy sauce, *mirin* and *sake*, and caster sugar to season, and bring to the boil. Check the seasoning and adjust with the white pepper and salt as necessary. Add the potato starch to thicken the sauce, and mix until the beef and the vegetables are well coated. Remove from the heat and sprinkle the *sansho* pepper on top.

5. Serve hot on a bed of rocket leaves. Garnish with the diced tomato.

Quality Points

- The beef should be tender and moist. It should have the flavour of the soy sauce and *mirin* and a hint of the *sansho*.

Chef's Tip

- *Sansho* adds heat and a citrus tanginess to the dish.

Measurements	Ingredients
400 g	Beef, topside or sirloin, cut into 1 cm slices
4 tbsp	Vegetable oil
1	Aubergine, quartered and cut into 3 cm chunks
1	Green pepper, halved, de-seeded and cut into 3 cm strips
2 tbsp	Japanese soy sauce
1 tbsp	*Mirin*
1 tbsp	*Sake*
1 tsp	Caster sugar
	Salt and ground white pepper to taste
1 tsp	Potato starch mixed with 1 tbsp of water
Pinch	Ground *sansho* pepper
Marinade	
2½ tbsp	Japanese soy sauce
1½ tbsp	*Mirin*
¼ tsp	Ground *sansho* pepper
Pinch	Bicarbonate of soda
1 tbsp	Water
Garnish	
50 g	Rocket leaves
2	Tomatoes, skinned, de-seeded and cut into 1 cm dice

Sukiyaki すき焼き

This dish is cooked at the table. You will need a tabletop burner and a sukiyaki skillet or shallow cast-iron pan.

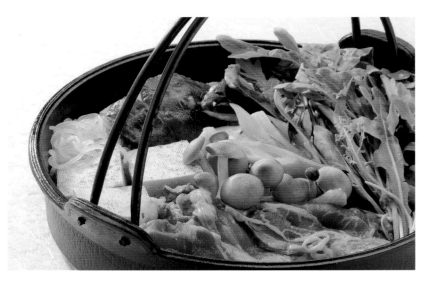

Preparation

- Cut the spring onions diagonally into 3 cm-thick slices.

- Blanch the *shira-taki* for 5 minutes, drain and refresh in cold water. Cut into 5 cm lengths

- Cut the grilled tofu into 4cm squares.

- Pull leaves off the *shun-giku*. Discard the stalks.

- Combine the ingredients for the *wari-shita* sauce.

- Arrange the sliced beef and other ingredients on a large platter ready to serve.

Method

1. Heat the *sukiyaki* skillet on the tabletop burner. Put the beef suet in the skillet and render the fat to lubricate the pan. Add quarter of the beef and spread it thinly over the surface of the skillet. Pour in the *wari-shita* sauce, just enough to cover the bottom of the pan.

Measurements	Ingredients
500 g	Beef, sirloin, cut into 2 mm slices
30 g	Fresh beef suet
4	Thick spring onions
200 g	Grilled tofu
200 g	*Shira-taki* (see p. 67)
300 g	*Shun-giku* (edible chrysanthemum) leaves (use rocket leaves if not available)
200 g	Cooked *udon* noodles (see p. 62)
Wari-shita sauce	
100 ml	Japanese soy sauce
30 g	Caster sugar
100 ml	*Mirin*
Condiments	
4	Eggs, very fresh

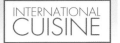

2. Place half the spring onions, the tofu squares and the *shira-taki* threads in the skillet, and turn down the heat to a simmer. After the tofu and *shira-taki* have absorbed some of the stock, add the *shun-giku* leaves (or rocket leaves).

3. When the leaves are slightly wilted, the *sukiyaki* is ready to be eaten. Take care not to overcook the beef slices or *shun-giku* leaves (the latter will get bitter).

4. Each diner takes an egg, breaks it into an individual bowl and beats it lightly.

5. All diners help themselves to the foods from the skillet as soon as they are cooked, dipping them into the beaten egg before eating.

6. Replenish the skillet with the remaining vegetables and beef as required. Pour in more *wari-shita* sauce or hot water, adjust the seasoning and repeat the above procedure.

7. Add the *udon* noodles at the end to soak up the reduced stock and eat to round off the meal.

Quality Points

- Take care not to overcook the ingredients, particularly the beef and *shun-giku* leaves.

Chef's Tip

- This is a dish made for appreciating high-quality meat. There are many regional variations of the seasoning.

Chicken and Egg on Steamed Rice
親子どんぶり

This dish is called *Oyako Donburi* in Japanese, or 'mother and child reunion'. (Approximately two cups of uncooked rice make four cups of cooked rice.)

Method

1. Cut the chicken into 2 cm pieces.

2. Make four individual portions of beaten egg.

3. Put all the ingredients for the stock in a pan and bring to the boil. Sieve the stock through muslin and divide into four portions.

4. In a small shallow pan, put one portion each of the stock, chicken, onion and *shiitake* mushrooms, and bring to the boil. Simmer until the chicken is cooked.

5. Sprinkle some of the spring onion on the above ingredients and pour the beaten egg over the top. Leave it for 20–30 seconds to allow the egg to set, and then garnish with the remaining spring onion.

6. Place one portion of the rice in each *donburi*-style bowl with a lid, transfer the chicken/egg mixture on top and replace the lid.

7. Serve piping hot so that the aroma of the chicken and egg wafts out when the lid is lifted.

Quality Points

- The egg should be just cooked, not runny.

Chef's Tip

- This is a typical light lunch, useful for using up any leftover chicken.

Measurements	Ingredients
150 g	Chicken leg (skinned and boned)
4	Eggs
4	Reconstituted dry shiitake mushrooms, cut into thin slices
50 g	Onion, cut into 1 mm-thick half-rounds
4 cups	Hot cooked Japanese rice
Stock	
400 ml	Water
4 tbsp	Japanese soy sauce
4 tbsp	*Mirin*
2½ tbsp	Caster sugar
5 g	*Hana-gatsuo* (bonito flakes)
5 cm	Dried *konbu*
Garnish	
1	Spring onion, cut into fine julienne (strips)

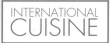

Glutinous Rice with Adzuki Beans 赤飯

This is traditionally served as part of a festive meal.

Method

1. Put the beans in a pan, add enough water to cover them and bring slowly to the boil. Discard the cooked liquid, replace with 600 ml of fresh water and bring to the boil again. Reduce the heat to a simmer and continue to cook until the beans are just done (about 30–45 minutes). Leave to cool down completely.

2. Drain the cooked beans but save the liquid.

3. Soak the rice in the saved reddish liquid for 1 hour. The rice will expand and turn pink, taking on the colour of the liquid.

Measurements	Ingredients
50 g	Adzuki beans, soaked overnight
380 ml	Cooking liquid from the adzuki beans, put aside
400 ml	Glutinous rice, washed
Garnish	
1 tbsp	Toasted black sesame seeds
1 tsp	Toasted salt

4. Place the soaked rice and cooked beans in a bowl and steam for 20–25 minutes.

5. When the rice is cooked, fluff it up with a rice paddle or fork.

6. Serve in individual rice bowls sprinkled with a mixture of the toasted black sesame seeds and salt.

Quality Points

- Care should be taken to ensure that the beans do not break while being simmered. The rice should be sticky but firm, and pink.

Chef's Tip

- If the saved liquid is insufficient to cover the rice, add water to make up the shortfall.

Grilled Teriyaki Chicken on Rice (Kiji Don) きじ丼

Method

1. Cut the chicken into pieces 4 cm wide and 1 cm thick.

2. Combine all the ingredients for the marinade and mix well.

3. Marinate the chicken for 30 minutes.

4. Grill the chicken on both sides, basting it with the marinade. When cooked, take it away from the heat and keep warm.

5. Reduce the marinade until it thickens.

6. Brush the spring onion pieces with oil and sprinkle with salt. Grill them until they wilt, taking care not burn them. Keep them warm.

7. Place one portion of the hot steamed rice in each *donburi*-style bowl with a lid. First, arrange the spring onions on the rice, then lay the chicken pieces on top and decorate with *nori* strips placed in a latticework pattern on top. Spoon over the reduced marinade and sprinkle on a pinch of ground *sansho* pepper. Replace the lid.

8. Serve very hot so that the aroma of the *sansho* and sauce wafts out when the lid is lifted.

Chef's Tip

• *Teriyaki* chicken can be used for this dish.

Measurements	Ingredients
300 g	Chicken leg (boned with skin)
4	Spring onions, cut into 5 cm lengths
2 tbsp	Vegetable oil
	Salt, to sprinkle
4 cups	Hot steamed rice
Marinade	
3 tbsp	*Mirin*
4 tbsp	Japanese soy sauce
1 tbsp	Caster sugar
Garnish	
½ sheet	*Nori* seaweed, cut into 3 cm-wide strips
Condiments	
Pinch	Ground *sansho* pepper

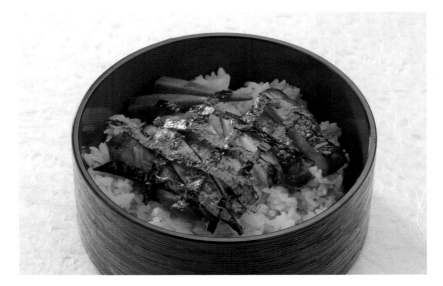

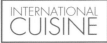

Deep-fried Breadcrumbed Pork Cutlets on Rice (Katsu-don) カツ丼

Preparations

- Follow the *tonkatsu* recipe on p. 158 up to step 6 and make four *tonkatsu*. Cut each *tonkatsu* into 2 cm-thick slices and keep warm.
- Divide the sliced onions and spring onions into four equal portions.
- Place all the ingredients for the sauce in a pan and bring to the boil. Remove from the heat and divide into four equal portions.

Method

1. Add one portion each of the onion slices and the sauce into a pan, bring to the boil and cook until the onions become transparent. Then add one portion of sliced *tonkatsu*.

2. Bring to the boil and pour in the beaten egg in a thin stream over the onion slices. Then, sprinkle spring onion.

3. Cover and turn the heat down to a simmer. Cook for 30 seconds until the egg sets. Do not let the egg get hard and dry.

4. Arrange a portion of the steamed rice in a *donburi*-style bowl with a lid and place a single portion of *tonkatsu* slices neatly on top. Transfer the egg and onion mixture to the bowl, pour the sauce over the top and put the lid back on.

5. Serve piping hot so that the *tonkatsu* and egg aroma wafts out when the lid is lifted.

Measurements	Ingredients
50 g	Onion, cut into 5 mm half-moon slices
4	*Tonkatsu* (see recipe on p. 158)
4	Eggs, each one individually beaten
4 cups	Hot cooked Japanese rice
Garnish	
4	Spring onions, cut into julienne (strips)
Sauce	
400 ml	*Dashi* stock
100 ml	*Mirin*
100 ml	Japanese soy sauce
2 tbsp	Caster sugar

Quality Points

- This dish should be served hot. The rice should be sticky but firm.

Chief's Tip

- This is a popular lunch in Japan and can be made with leftover *tonkatsu*. Make it just before serving to prevent it getting soggy. A chicken cutlet can be used instead of pork.

Rice with Three-coloured Toppings (Chicken, Salmon and Egg on Rice) 三色ご飯

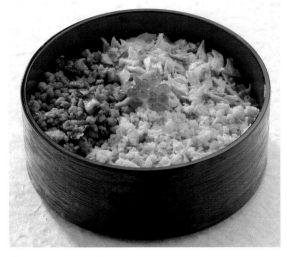

Measurements	Ingredients
4 cups	Hot steamed Japanese rice
Chicken topping	
250 g	Chicken, finely minced
6	Shiitake mushrooms, stalks removed and cut into 1 cm dice
2 tbsp	Vegetable oil
3 tbsp	*Sake*
1 tbsp	Japanese soy sauce
½ tsp	Ginger, finely grated
Salmon topping	
200 g	Salmon fillet
Salmon marinade	
100 ml	*Sake*
100 ml	Japanese soy sauce
2 tbsp	Caster sugar
Egg topping	
4	Eggs, beaten
1 tbsp	Caster sugar
1 tbsp	Japanese light soy Sauce
¼ tsp	Salt
1 tbsp	*Sake*
Sauce for rice	
200 ml	*Dashi* stock
3 tbsp	Japanese soy sauce
½ tbsp	Caster sugar
Garnish	
2 tsp	Salmon roe

Preparation

• Rinse the salmon in cold water and dry. Mix together the ingredients for the salmon marinade, making sure the sugar is completely dissolved. Marinate the salmon for 1–2 hours.

• Trim the chicken and food-process to make fine chicken mince.

• Cook two cups of rice to make four cups of steamed rice.

Method

1. Pour the vegetable oil into a pan and stir-fry the minced chicken and mushrooms. Increase to a high heat, stirring constantly to keep the chicken pieces separated until they resemble breadcrumbs in appearance. Add all seasonings except the ginger. When the chicken is cooked and the liquid has almost evaporated, mix in the ginger. Transfer to a colander to drain completely and cool.

2. Remove the salmon from the marinade and pat dry. Grill it until cooked and slightly browned. Put it aside to cool, then flake the flesh to the size of pumpkin seeds.

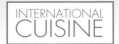

3. Mix together the beaten eggs, sugar, light soy sauce, salt and *sake*, and make fine, but well-cooked, scrambled eggs.

4. In a small pan, mix the rice sauce ingredients. Bring to the boil and simmer for 1–2 minutes. Remove from the heat and keep warm.

5. To assemble, put each portion of hot rice into an individual *donburi*-style bowl (or Japanese style lunchbox) with a lid. Pour 2–3 tbsp of the hot sauce over the rice to moisten it. Divide the rice surface equally into three segments and cover each with one of the three toppings. Garnish the centre with ½ tsp of salmon roe.

Chef's Tip

- You can use any leftover grilled or *teriyaki* salmon as a topping.

Steamed Seasoned Rice with Chicken and Vegetables

かやく ご飯

This is a very popular rice dish. The quantity of liquid is compensated for by the natural moisture in the ingredients and marinade.

Method

1. Wash the rice in a bowl under the tap, changing the water several times until it runs clear.

2. Drain the rice in a sieve and leave for 30 minutes.

3. Blanch the frozen peas by soaking them in boiling water for 30 seconds and then drain.

4. Mix together all the ingredients for the marinade. Marinate the chicken and *age* for 15 minutes and then drain.

5. Combine all the ingredients for the stock. Place the rice and all the other ingredients, except the peas, in a heavy-bottomed medium-sized pan with a lid, or a rice cooker, and pour on the stock. Put the lid on and cook following the steamed rice recipe (on p. 79).

Measurements	Ingredients
3 cups (600 ml)	Japanese rice
40 g	Frozen peas
20 g	Carrots, cut into 1 cm dice
3	Reconstituted dried shiitake mushrooms, excess moisture squeezed out and cut into 1 cm squares
½ sheet	*Age* (deep-fried bean curd), cut into 1 cm squares
60 g	Chicken leg meat, cut into 3 cm dice
½ sheet	*Konnyaku*, cut into 1 cm dice
Stock	
720 ml	*Dashi* stock
½ tsp	Salt
2 tbsp	Dark soy sauce
1 tbsp	*Sake*
Marinade	
3 tbsp	Japanese light soy sauce
1 tbsp	*Sake*
1 tbsp	*Mirin*

6. When the liquid is absorbed, turn off the heat. Allow the pan to sit on the stove undisturbed for 5 minutes.

7. Take the lid off and add the blanched peas. Mix in using a rice paddle and fluff up the rice.

Chef's Tip

• This rice can be used as a stuffing for seasoned tofu pouches (*Inari-zushi*, see recipe on p. 103) in place of sushi rice. Be sure to cool the rice first.

Tea-flavoured Steamed Rice 茶飯

Method

1. Wash the rice under cold water until the water runs clear. Drain.

2. Boil the water and put the teabags in to make tea. Add the salt.

3. Cook the rice with the tea following the steamed rice recipe on p. 79.

4. When the rice is cooked, fluff it up as in the above recipe.

Measurements	Ingredients
2 cups (400 ml)	Japanese rice
450 ml	Water
2	Japanese *bancha* or *hojicha* teabags
½ tsp	Salt

Quality Points

• Rice should be sticky but firm, and the grains should not be squashed.

Chef's Tip

• This rice goes very well with vegetarian dishes.

Tempura on Rice 天丼

Approximately two cups of uncooked rice make four cups of cooked rice.

Method

1. Make *tempura* by following the recipe on p. 128. Keep warm.

2. In a small pan combine all the ingredients for the sauce and bring to the boil. Simmer for 2 minutes.

Measurements	Ingredients
4 cups	Hot cooked Japanese rice
4 portions	Vegetable/white fish fillet/seafood/*tempura*
Sauce	
250 ml	*Dashi* stock
4 tbsp	Japanese soy sauce
4 tbsp	*Sake*
2 tbsp	Caster sugar

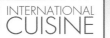
3. Put a single portion of hot rice in an individual *donburi*-style bowl with a lid. On top, arrange one serving of hot *tempura*. Pour 2 or 3 tablespoonsful of the hot sauce over the *tempura* and the rice, and replace the lid.

4. Serve piping hot so that the aroma of *tempura* and sauce wafts out when the lid is lifted.

Quality Points

- The *tempura* should be light and not oily. The rice should be sticky but firm.

Chef's Tips

- This is the best way to use up any leftover *tempura*. It makes a very good lunch dish.

Cold Soba Noodles with Dipping Sauce
ざる蕎麦

Method

1. Combine all the ingredients for the dipping sauce in a pan and bring to the boil. Remove the *konbu* when the sauce starts to boil. Simmer to reduce the liquid to 80 per cent. Sieve the stock through muslin and leave it to cool.

2. Cook the dried *soba* noodles al dente in boiling water, following the instructions on the packet. As soon as they are cooked, drain and plunge the noodles in cold water, then run under the tap to remove any surface starch.

3. Drain well. Arrange each cold *soba* portion on a bamboo serving sieve and sprinkle the *nori* seaweed strips on top. Chill.

4. Pour each portion of dipping sauce into an individual cup and arrange the condiments on a small side plate.

5. Serve the *soba* very cold with the condiments.

Measurements	Ingredients
440 g	Dried *soba* noodles
Dipping sauce	
75 ml	Soy sauce
45 ml	*Mirin*
300 ml	Water
1 tbsp	Caster sugar
10 cm square	Dried *konbu*
10 g	Bonito flakes
Garnish	
1 sheet	*Nori* sheets, cut into 5 mm strips
Condiments	
1 tsp	*Wasabi* paste
1	Spring onion, very thinly sliced

Variation

Cold *soba* noodles with tempura: serve hot *tempura* on the side, with the *soba* and the dipping sauce.

Quality Points

* *Soba* noodles should be cooked al dente.

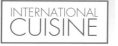
Chef's Tip

- The sauce will improve if made in advance. It will keep for several days in the fridge. Suitable additional condiments are toasted sesame seeds and grated *daikon* radish (mooli).

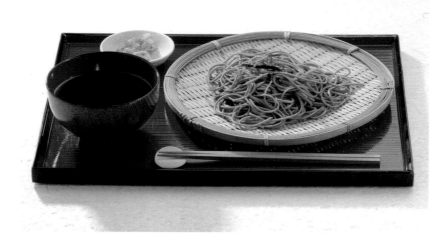

Soup Soba Noodles with Chicken 鶏蕎麦

Method

1. Combine all the ingredients for the stock in a pan and bring to the boil. When it comes to the boil, remove the *konbu*. Continue to simmer for a further 2 minutes. Sieve the stock through muslin.

2. Reheat the stock in a clean pan and poach the chicken pieces.

3. Cook the dried *soba* noodles in boiling water making sure they remain al dente. Plunge them in cold water to cool. Remove any surface starch in running water and drain well.

4. Place each portion of the *soba* in boiling water until it is heated through and then drain. Arrange the *soba* in individual warm *donburi*-style bowls. Place a single portion of chicken and spring onions on top of each.

Measurements	Ingredients
440 g	Dried *soba* noodles
150 g	Chicken breast, cut into 2 cm slices
Stock	
140 ml	Soy sauce
75 ml	*Mirin*
1½ litre	Water
10 cm square	Dried *konbu*
50 g	Bonito flakes
Condiments	
1 tsp	*Shichimi* pepper
Garnish	
1	Spring onion, very thinly sliced

5. Bring the stock to the boil and pour it over the soba so that it is covered.

6. Serve piping hot with *shichimi* pepper as a condiment on the side.

Variation

Tempura soba noodles: use a single portion of *tempura* instead of the chicken in step 4.

Quality Points

* *Soba* should be cooked al dente. The stock should be clear, light in colour and not cloudy.

Chef's Tip

* Warm the *soba* swiftly in the boiling water so that it will not lose its al dente texture.

Soup Udon Noodle with Simmered Bean Curd きつねうどん

Method

1. Boil the *age* (fried bean curd) in plenty of hot water for 1 minute and discard the water. Add just enough fresh boiling water to cover the blanched *age* and simmer for 4–5 minutes with a drop-lid on top.

2. Add the sugar and continue to cook for 5 minutes. Add the soy sauce and reduce the liquid to one-third. Leave to cool.

3. Place all the ingredients for the stock in a pan and bring to the boil. When the stock comes to the boil, reduce the heat to a simmer and continue to cook for 6 minutes. Sieve the liquid through muslin.

4. Cook the dried *udon* noodles in boiling water making sure that they remain al dente. Drain and plunge them in cold water to cool. Remove any starch in running water and drain well.

5. Place each portion of *udon* in boiling water until it is heated through. Drain and arrange each portion in a warm *donburi*-style bowl. Place a few slices of simmered bean curd and spring onions on top of each portion.

Measurements	Ingredients
440 g	Dried *udon* noodles
Stock	
75 ml	Light soy sauce
45 ml	*Mirin*
1½ litres	Water
10 cm square	Dried *konbu*
30 g	Bonito flakes
Simmered bean curd	
4 sheets	*Age* (fried bean curd)
3½ tbsp	Caster sugar
2½ tbsp	Soy sauce
Condiments	
1 tsp	*Shichimi* pepper
Garnish	
1	Spring onion, very thinly sliced

6. Bring the soup to the boil and pour it over the *udon* until it is well covered.

7. Serve hot with *shichimi* pepper as a condiment on the side.

Variation

***Tempura udon* noodles:** use two pieces of prawn tempura in place of the bean curd in step 5.

Quality Points

- *Udon* should be cooked so that it remains al dente. The stock should be clear and light in colour.

Chef's Tip

- Warm the *udon* only briefly in boiling water so that it will not cook further. Light soy sauce gives the stock its unique colour.

Cold Somen Noodles with Dipping Sauce
冷やしそうめん

This is a delicious dish for a hot summer's day.

Method

1. Combine all the ingredients for the dipping sauce in a pan and bring to the boil. Lower the heat to a simmer and bring to the boil again. Leave aside to cool. Strain the stock through muslin and then refrigerate.

2. Cook the dried *somen* noodles in boiling water, following the instructions on the packet. As soon as they are cooked, drain them and plunge in cold water. Run them under the tap to remove any surface starch. Drain well.

3. Arrange each portion of cold *somen* in an individual glass bowl containing ice cubes.

4. Pour each portion of the dipping sauce into an individual sauce cup and the arrange condiments on small side plates.

5. Serve the *somen* cold with the condiments on the side.

Measurements	Ingredients
440 g	Dried *somen* noodles
Dipping sauce	
60 ml	Soy sauce
60 ml	*Mirin*
300 ml	Water
20 g	Bonito flakes
Condiments	
20 g	Ginger, finely grated
4	Spring onions, very thinly sliced

Quality Points

- *Somen* noodles should be cooked so that they remain al dente. The sauce should taste slightly sweet.

Chef's Tip

- The sauce will improve if made in advance. It will keep for several days in the fridge.

Cold Hiyamugi Noodles with Dipping Sauce 冷やしひやむぎ

Another delicious dish for a hot summer's day.

Method

1. Place all the ingredients for the dipping sauce in a pan and bring to the boil. Lower the heat to a simmer and then bring to the boil again. Leave aside to cool. Sieve the cooled sauce through muslin and then refrigerate.

2. Cook the dried *hiyamugi* noodles in boiling water following the instructions on the packet. As soon as they are cooked, drain them and plunge in cold water. Remove any surface starch by running them under the tap. Drain well.

3. Arrange each portion of cold *hiyamugi* in an individual glass bowl containing ice cubes.

4. Pour each portion of the dipping sauce into an individual dipping sauce cup and arrange the condiments on small side plates.

5. Serve the *hiyamugi* cold with the condiments.

Measurements	Ingredients
440 g	Dried *hiyamugi* noodles
Dipping sauce	
60 ml	Soy sauce
60 ml	*Mirin*
300 ml	Water
20 g	Bonito flakes
Condiments	
20 g	Ginger, finely grated
4	Spring onions, very thinly sliced

Quality Points

- *Hiyamugi* noodles should be cooked so that they remain al dente. The sauce should have a sweet overtone.

Chef's Tip

- The sauce will taste better if made in advance. It will keep for several days in the fridge.

To supplement those in this chapter, you will find more soup recipes in Chapter 9, 'Getting started: beginners' recipes'.

Daikon Radish and Fried Bean Curd Miso Soup 大根と揚げの味噌汁

Preparation

- Blanch the *age* sheet in boiling water for 1–2 minutes to remove the surface oil, and then drain. Cut the sheet in half lengthways and slice into 5 mm julienne (strips).

Method

1. Pour the *dashi* stock into a pan. Add the *daikon* radish and *age*, and bring to the boil. Simmer for 5–6 minutes, removing any scum until the *daikon* is cooked.

2. Dissolve the miso in a ladleful of the stock and then mix into the soup. Bring to the boil.

3. Adjust the seasoning to taste and add the rocket leaves just before removing from the heat.

4. Ladle the soup into individual bowls and sprinkle on a pinch of the *shichimi* pepper just before serving.

Measurements	Ingredients
800 ml	*Dashi* stock
150 g	*Daikon* radish (mooli), peeled and cut into 4 cm julienne (strips)
1 sheet	*Age* (fried bean curd)
30 g	Miso
50 g	Rocket leaves
Condiments	
Pinch	*Shichimi* pepper

Quality Points

- *Daikon* radish and *age* should be cooked so that they remain al dente. The soup should be a harmonious blend of miso and *dashi* stock, and not salty.

Pork and Vegetable Miso Soup 薩摩汁

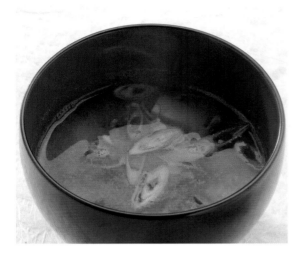

Measurements	Ingredients
300 g	Pork shoulder
1 litre	Water
50 g	Carrots
100 g	*Daikon* radish (mooli)
100 g	*Sato-imo* (eddoe)
40 g	White miso
25 g	Miso
4	Shiitake mushrooms, stalks removed and cut into 1 cm slices
2	Spring onions, finely sliced
Condiments	
Pinch	*Shichimi* pepper

Preparation

- Peel the *sato-imo* (eddoe) tubers thickly and cut into 5 mm slices. Soak in water to prevent discolouration.
- Trim the pork and cut into 3 cm cubes.
- Peel the *daikon* radish (mooli) and carrots. Cut into quarters and then into 5 mm slices.

Method

1. Put the pork and water in a pan and bring to the boil. Continue to cook over a low heat for 15 minutes.

2. Add the carrots, *daikon* radish and *sato-imo* to the stock and cook until they are just done. Test for 'doneness' with a knife point or skewer.

3. Dissolve the miso in a ladleful of the stock – one type of miso at a time – and mix it in. Adjust the seasoning, and add the mushrooms and spring onions. Bring to the boil once.

4. Ladle the soup into individual bowls and sprinkle each portion with a pinch of the *shichimi* pepper. Serve immediately.

Quality Points

- The soup should be free of miso lumps and the vegetables should be cooked so that they remain al dente.

Sesame-flavoured Miso Soup with Vegetables and Tofu けんちん汁

This hearty soup is a mixture of ingredients with different textures.

Preparation

- Wrap the tofu in a teacloth and place a clean chopping board on top to add weight. Leave aside for 30 minutes to squeeze out excess water.

- Cut the *age* in half lengthways and slice into 2 cm strips.

- Peel the *sato-imo* (eddoe tuber) and rub with salt to remove any sliminess. Cut into 3 cm-thick slices and soak in water to prevent discolouration.

- Peel and quarter the *daikon* radish (mooli) and cut into 5 mm-thick slices.

- Cut the carrots into 2.5 cm thick rounds (see vegetable cuts on p. 28).

- Sprinkle salt over the *konnyaku* and soften it by pounding on it a few times with a rolling pin. Rinse off the salt in warm water. Tear it into 1 cm pieces and dry-toast in a pan until the excess moisture evaporates.

- Wash the burdock, scrape off the skin and roll-cut into 1 cm wedges (see vegetable cuts on p. 29).

Measurements	Ingredients
100 g	*Daikon* radish (mooli)
100 g	*Sato-imo* (eddoe)
30 g	Burdock (optional)
100 g	Carrots
2 tbsp	Sesame oil
1 sheet	*Age* (fried bean curd)
1 sheet	*Konnyaku*
800 ml	*Dashi* stock
250 g	Tofu
80 g	Miso
	Salt, sufficient to sprinkle over the *konnyaku*
1 tsp	Ginger, finely grated
2	Spring onions, thinly sliced

Method

1. Blanch each vegetable in boiling water, drain and leave aside.

2. Heat the sesame oil in a pan and sauté the *sato-imo* (eddoe). Add the *age* (fried bean curd), carrots, *daikon* radish and *konnyaku*, in that order, until they absorb the sesame flavour.

3. Add the *dashi* stock and cook until the *sato-imo* is almost done. Tear the tofu by hand into 3 cm pieces and add to the soup. Heat the soup slowly until it comes almost to the boil. Dissolve the miso in a ladleful of the soup and then mix it in.

4. Adjust the seasoning to taste. Add the spring onion slices and grated ginger, and bring to the boil just once.

5. Ladle the soup into individual bowls and serve very hot.

Quality Points

- The vegetables should be cooked so that they remain al dente, and the miso completely dissolved.

Chef's Tip

- Try not to bring the soup to the boil repeatedly, as the miso will lose its flavour. *Sato-imo* (eddoe) is available from Asian and Caribbean grocers in the UK.

Daikon Radish in Yuzu Sweet Vinegar
柚子大根

Method

1. Combine all the ingredients for the sweet vinegar and simmer gently over a low heat to dissolve the sugar completely. Leave to cool.

2. When the vinegar is cold, add the *daikon* batons and the *yuzu* rind, and leave for 3–4 hours before serving.

Quality Points

- *Daikon* should be crunchy. It should taste sweet and sour with a hint of citrus flavour.

Chef's Tip

- This dish can be stored in a container in the fridge for up to five or six days.

Measurements	Ingredients
20 cm	*Daikon* radish (mooli), peeled and cut into 1 cm x 1 cm x 5 cm rectangles
1	*Yuzu* citron (if unavailable, use lime or tangerine) rind, finely grated
Sweet vinegar	
120 ml	Japanese rice vinegar
200 ml	Water
80 g	Caster sugar
2 tsp	Salt

Pickled Chinese Cabbage 白菜の山椒漬け

Method

1. Cut the Chinese cabbage leaves and stalks separately into strips 2 cm x 5 cm wide.

2. Mix the *Sichuan* peppercorns into the cabbage strips.

3. Rub the salt into the cabbage and peppercorns, and mix well. Leave to stand for 4–8 hours.

4. Combine the ingredients for the sweet vinegar, making sure the sugar is dissolved completely. If necessary, gently heat the vinegar.

5. Squeeze the water out of the cabbage and pour cooled sweet vinegar over it. Leave for 2–3 hours.

6. Serve as pickles in a small serving dish.

Quality Points

- The cabbage should be crunchy and taste sweet and sour with a hint of citrus flavour.

Chef's Tip

- This dish can be stored in an airtight container in the fridge for 5–6 days.

Measurements	Ingredients
500 g	Chinese cabbage leaves
1 tbsp	*Sichuan* peppercorns
1 tbsp	Salt
Sweet vinegar	
100 ml	Japanese rice vinegar
4 tbsp	Caster sugar
Garnish	
3 cm	Ginger, shredded and soaked in water

Sweet and Sour Cabbage and Cucumber
キャベツのもみ漬け

Method

1. Place all the vegetables and the dried chilli into a large bowl, sprinkle with the salt and mix well. Leave for 10 minutes.

2. Add the sugar, vinegar and sesame oil, and rub in with both hands. Leave for another 5 minutes.

3. Squeeze out as much water as possible before serving.

4. This dish can be served as a salad or pickles.

Quality Points

- All the vegetables should be crunchy, and should taste slightly hot and sour.

Chef's Tip

- This dish can be stored in an airtight container in the fridge for 5–7 days.

Measurements	Ingredients
½	Cucumber, de-seeded and cut into 2–3 cm batons
1	Carrot, peeled and shredded
500 g	Tenderpoint cabbage, stalks removed and cut into 3 cm squares
1–2	Dried chilli, de-seeded and cut into 1 cm rounds
2 tsp	Salt
2 tbsp	Sugar
3 tbsp	Japanese rice vinegar
1 tsp	Sesame oil

Adzuki Bean Dessert ぜんざい

Methods

1. Wash the soaked beans under cold running water and discard any broken pieces.

2. Transfer the beans to a pan and add enough water to cover. Bring slowly to the boil.

3. Discard the red-coloured liquid. Pour in fresh cold water and bring to the boil again.

Measurements	Ingredients
300 g	Dried *adzuki* beans, soaked overnight
125 g	Caster sugar
Pinch	Salt

4. Reduce the heat to a simmer and cook until the beans are just done, which should take about 30–45 minutes. Keep skimming off any scum while simmering.

5. Cover the pan and remove from the heat. Leave aside for 1 hour.

6. Put the pan on a low heat and bring the beans back to the boil. Reduce the heat to a simmer, add the sugar and continue to cook for about 10 minutes. Leave to stand for 1–2 hours, or overnight for a thicker consistency and richer flavour.

7. Reheat the beans. Taste to check sweetness and add a pinch of salt, which will intensify the sweetness.

8. A standard portion size is about 100 ml. Serve in individual bowls, either hot or cold.

Chef's Tip

- As this dish is high in sugar, it can be frozen. One or two grilled mochi (sticky Japanese rice cakes, see p. 49) per person can be added at the end of step 7 and the dish served as a snack.

Green Tea (*Matcha*) Ice Cream
抹茶アイスクリーム

Method

1. Dissolve the *matcha* (powdered green tea) in hot water and leave to stand for 15 minutes.

2. Bring the milk to the boil. Take it off the heat and add the green tea.

3. Cream the egg yolks and sugar in a bowl until very pale.

4. Continue whisking, add the milky tea and mix well.

5. Pour the above into a clean pan and place on to a low heat. Stir continuously with a wooden spoon until the mixture thickens and coats the back of the spoon. Take care not to overheat the mixture.

6. Strain the custard using a fine-meshed strainer. Cool to room temperature, stirring occasionally to release the heat. Add the double cream and mix well. Transfer to an airtight container and refrigerate for 6 hours or overnight.

7. Pour into an ice cream maker and churn-freeze. When ready, remove and store at −20°C.

8. To serve, arrange one scoop with poached pink grapefruit segments in each individual bowl with sesame tuilles if desired.

Measurements	Ingredients
10 g	*Matcha* (powdered Japanese green tea)
50 ml	Hot water
200 ml	Milk
5	Egg yolks
100 g	Caster sugar
150ml	Double cream
Garnish	
	Pink grapefruit segments, poached
	Sesame tuilles (optional)

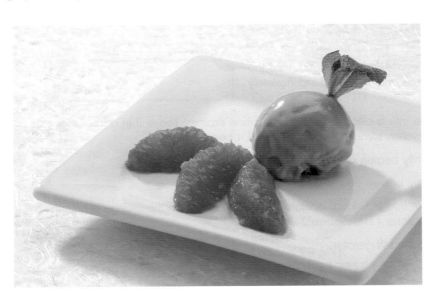

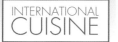

JA Centre (Tazaki Foods)
Unit B
Eley Industrial Estate
Eley Road
London N18 3BH
Tel: 020 8803 8942

Japan Centre Food Shop
212 Piccadilly
London W1 9HG
Tel: 020 7434 4218

J-mart
Oriental City
399 Edgware Road
London NW9 0JJ
Tel: 020 8205 3988

Marimo
350–356 Regent's Park Road
Finchley
London N3 2LJ
Tel: 020 8346 1042

Natural Natural (Ealing Common)
20 Station Parade
Uxbridge Road
London W5 3LD
Tel: 020 8992 0770

Natural Natural (Finchley Road)
1 Goldhurst Terrace
London NW6 3HX
Tel: 020 7624 5734

New Loon Moon
9A Gerrard Street
London W1D 5PN
Tel: 020 7734 3887

Oriental City
399 Edgware Road
Colindale
London NW9 0JJ
Tel/Fax: 020 8200 0848

Rice Wine Shop
82 Brewer Street
London W1
Tel: 020 7439 3705

TK Trading
Unit 6–7 The Chase Centre
Chase Road
London NW10 6QD
Tel: 020 8453 1743

Wing Yip (London)
395 Edgware Road
Cricklewood
London NW2 6LN
Tel: 020 8450 0422

Outside London

Birmingham
Wing Yip
375 Nechells Road
Nechells
Birmingham B7 5NT
Tel: 0121 327 3838
Fax: 0121 327 6612

Brighton
Midori
19 Marlborough Place
Brighton
East Sussex
Tel: 01273 601460
Fax: 01273 620422

Cambridge
Seoul Plaza 3
91–93 Mill Road
Cambridge CB1 2AB
Tel: 01223 303610

Canterbury
Sky Door
60A Northgate
Canterbury
Kent CT1 1BB
Tel: 01227 784200

Croydon

Wing Yip
550 Purley Way
Croydon
Surrey CR0 3RF
Tel: 020 8688 4880

Kingston upon Thames

Miura Foods (Kingston)
44 Coombe Road
Kingston Upon Thames
Surrey
Tel: 020 8549 8076

Ledbury

Ceci Paolo The Delicatessen
21 High Street
Ledbury
Herefordshire HR8 1DS
Tel: 01531 632976

Manchester

Hang Won Hong
Connaught Building
58–60 George Street
Manchester M1 4HF
Tel: 0161 228 6182

Wing Yip
Oldham Road
Ancoats
Manchester M4 5HU
Tel: 0161 832 3215

Samsi Express
Basement
36–38 Whitworth Street
Manchester M1 3NR
Tel: 0161 279 0023

New Malden

Seoul Plaza
36 High Street
New Malden
Surrey KT3 4HE
Tel: 020 8949 4329

Seoul Plaza 2
126 Maiden Road
New Malden
Surrey KT3 6DD
Tel: 020 8942 9552

Newcastle upon Tyne

Setsu Japan
196a Heaton Road
Newcastle upon Tyne
Tel: 0191 265 9970

Reading

Ayame
Unit L13
Gyosei College
Acacia Road
Reading
Berks
Tel: 01734 3106470

Swindon

Jasmin
Stanton House Hotel
The Avenue
Stanton Fitzwarren
Swindon
Wilts
Tel: 01793 861777

Mail-order organic Japanese

Clearspring Direct
Tel: 020 8746 0152
Fax: 020 8811 8893
email: mailorder@clearspring.co.uk
website: www.clearspring.co.uk

Index

page numbers in *italics* refer to illustrations

adzuki beans, with glutinous rice 17, 59, 168, 186
agar-agar 60
age (fried bean curd)
    with braised *hijiki* seaweed 106
    pouches with stuffed sushi rice 103–4, *103*
    soup with vegetables and tofu 182–3
    soup with *Daikon* radish 180
    with soup *udon* noodle 177–8
    with steamed rice and chicken 172–3
    uses of 50
amazu (sweet vinegar) dressing 42–3
antioxidants 14–15
arrowhead 51
asparagus 88–9, *88*
aubergines
    cutting techniques for *29*
    from Kyoto 7
    shallow-fried 113, *113*
    uses of 51
avocado, with *wasabi* dressing 112

bamboo shoots 52, 118–19, 142–3, *143*
bamboo sushi mat 23
barbecuing 25–6
bavarois, green tea with orange 188
bean curd *see age*; tofu
bean sprouts 52, 75
beans, French 117–18, *117*
    see also adzuki beans
beef
    braised (with potatoes) 155–6, *156*
    shabu-shabu (cooked at table) 161–2
    stir-fried with ground *sansho* pepper 164

sukiyaki (cooked at table) 165–6, *165*
tataki (beef sashimi) 154–5, *154*
    and tofu in sweet miso 105–6
beni-shoga (salted ginger) 66
bevelling cutting technique *29*
blowfish 9–10
bonito, dried fillets 61
breadcrumbs 61
Buddhist influence 5–6
burdock 52, 81, 142, 182–3

cabbage 184–5, *185*
California roll 9
caloric density pyramid 13, *15*
calorie content 12–14
cancer 11
cardiovascular disease 12
carrots
    with braised beef and potatoes 155–6, *156*
    with chicken 142–3, *143*
    cuts for 28
    from Kyoto 7
    pork and vegetable miso soup 181–2, *181*
    soup with vegetables and tofu 182–3
    with steamed rice and chicken 172–3
    stir-fried with chilli 81–2, *81*
cha soba noodles 63
charcoal barbecuing 26
chicken
    with braised Japanese vegetables 142–3, *143*
    broth 78–9, *78*
    and cucumber in vinegar dressing 115
    deep-fried breadcrumbed 143–4
    deep-fried goujons 145
    deep-fried marinated (*tatsuta-age*) 146–7, *146*

and egg on steamed rice 167
grilled spicy 148–9, *148*
minced balls (*tsukune*) 150
with salmon and egg on rice 171–2, *171*
savoury custard cup 125–6, *125*
on skewers (*yakitori*) 149–50, *149*
soup *soba* noodles with 176–7
steamed 151
with steamed rice and vegetables 172–3
stock 41
with stuffed lotus roots 152–3
stuffed shiitake mushrooms 151–2
teriyaki *1*, 18, 74–5, 168–9, *169*
chilli 81–2, *81*, 88–9, *88*
Chinese cabbage 184–5
Chinese garlic chives 52
Chinese leaves 52, 116–17, *116*
chives, Chinese garlic 52
cholesterol 15, 16, 17
chopsticks 23
chrysanthemum leaves (edible) 53
citrus rind pine needle *30*
cod
    deep-fried 135
    fillets en papillote 131–2, *132*
condiments 64–5
constipation 15
cooking methods
    barbecuing 25–6
    deep-frying 26–7
    grilling 25–6
    shallow-frying 26
    simmering 25
    steaming 27–8
    stir-frying 26
cucumber
    and cabbage (sweet and sour) 185
    and chicken in Japanese vinegar dressing 115

rolls 97–8
uses of 52–3
and *wakame* seaweed with Japanese vinegar dressing 76–7, *76*
custard cup 125–6, *125*
cutting techniques, decorative cuts 28–30

dai-dai citron 64
Daikon radish
    cuts for 28–9
    and fried bean curd miso soup 180
    with grilled marinated salmon 80–1, *80*
    pickle 184
    pork and vegetable miso soup 181–2, *181*
    salad 122
    sesame-flavoured miso soup with vegetables and tofu 182–3
    simmered with miso sauce 119–20, *120*
    in tofu and white miso sauce 110–11
    uses of 53
dashi stock, primary 38–41
decorative cutting technique *29–30*
deep-frying 24, 26–7
dessert
    adzuki beans 186
    green tea bavarois with orange segments 188
    green tea ice cream 186–7, *187*
devil's tongue jelly 15, 67
diabetes 15
dipping sauces 43, *43–4*
domyoji-ko powder 49
dressing
    miso 44
    vinegar 41–3
drop-in lid 25
duck, grilled marinated 147–8

eddoe 56, 181
eggs
    with chicken and salmon on rice 171–2, *171*

eggs *continued*
  and chicken on steamed
    rice 167
  cold poached egg starter
    123
  golden thread eggs 93
  Japanese rolled omelette
    123–4, *123*
  savoury custard cup
    125–6, *125*
  scattered sushi (Osaka
    style) 69, 72–3
  soft Japanese rolled
    omelette 126–7
  soup 73
  quails' eggs, sugarsnap
    peas and spring onions
    87–8, *87*
  sushi (omelette with
    mushrooms) 102–3,
    102
enokidake mushrooms 53,
  56

fan (cooling) 23
fatty fish 16
fermented foods 15
filleting
  flat fish *34*
  round fish *33*
  for *sashimi* 35–6
fish
  blowfish 9–10
  cakes 67
  filleting 33–6
  gutting 31–2
  health benefits of 16
  salt-baked white fish
    fillets 132–3
  salt-grilled 133–4, *133*
  savoury custard cup
    125–6, *125*
  scattered sushi (Osaka
    style) 69, 72–3
  simmered flat fish 134
  steamed white fish and
    tofu 140–1, *140*
  tempura 128–9, *129*,
    173–4
  see also cod; mackerel;
    prawns; salmon;
    sardines; *sashimi*;
    squid; trout; tuna
fish cleavers 22
French beans with crushed
  sesame seeds 117–18,
  117
frying *see* deep-frying;
  shallow-frying; stir-fries
fu (wheat gluten) 59–60
futomaki rolls 94–6, *95–6*

ganmodoki 5, 50
garlic 5

garlic chives 52
gas barbecuing 26
geography of Japan 3–4
gift-wrapping food 8
ginger
  salted (*beni-shoga*) 66
  sardines simmered with
    136
  sauce with pork loin
    160–1, *161*
  sauce with steamed
    chicken 151
  sauce with tofu steak
    and mushrooms 85,
    86
  stem 57
  uses of 53
ginger-flavoured soy sauce
  45
gingko nuts, uses of 54
glutinous rice 48–9, 168
gourd shavings 60
graters 22
green peppers 57
green soya beans 54
green tea
  bavarois with orange
    segments 188
  ice cream 186–7, *187*
grilling 25–6
ground sesame sauce 43–4
gutting techniques 31, *32*

hana-gatsuo 60
haute cuisine 5, 6
health properties
  adzuki beans 17
  antioxidants 14–15
  calorie content 12–14
  cancer 11
  cardiovascular disease 12
  cholesterol 15, 16, 17
  constipation 15
  diabetes 15
  fermented foods 15
  konnyaku (devil's tongue
    jelly) 15
  longevity 11
  menopause 11
  omega-3 fats 16
  power foods 15–17
  seaweed 16
  shiitake mushrooms 16
  soya beans 11–12, 15
herbs 58–9
hijiki seaweed 16, 60, 106
hiyamugi noodles 63, 179
honzen-ryori cuisine 5, 8

ice cream, green tea
  186–7, *187*
ichiban dashi (stock) 38–9
inaniwa udon noodles 62–3
ita-kamaboko 67

ito-kezuri 60
ito-konnyaku 66

jade rice 90, *90*
Japanese yam 54
joshin-ko powder 49

kabocha squash 54, 120–1,
  121
kaiseki cuisine 5, 6–8
kamaboko (fish cakes) 67
kanpyo (dried gourd
  shavings) 60, 93
kanten 60
kelp *see konbu*
kimpira carrots 81–2, *81*
kinako 51
kinome leaves 58
kishimen noodles 63
knives 21–2
komatsuna 54
konbu (kelp) 16, 39, 61
konnyaku (devil's tongue
  jelly) 15, 67
kuzu 66
Kyoto 3, 5, 6–7, 9

lacquer ware 6
lemon, cutting technique
  for *30*
longevity 11
lotus root 55, 152–3

mackerel
  in miso sauce 129–30,
    130
  sashimi 137–8, *138*
matsutake mushrooms 55
meat
  consumption of 10
  see also beef; pork
menopause 11
menu planning 18
mint 59
mirin 47
miso 44, 47–8
mitsuba leaves 58, *59*
mizuna 55
mooli *see Daikon* radish
mushrooms
  enokidake 53
  matsutake 55
  nameko 55
  shimeji 56–7
  with tofu steak and
    ginger sauce 85, 86
  wood ear 58
  see also shiitake mushrooms
mustard 64
mustard soy sauce 45
mustard spinach 54
mustard-flavoured miso
  dressing 44
myoga 55

nameko mushrooms 55
natto 15, 51
niban dashi (stock) 39–40
noodles
  with beef *shabu-shabu*
    161–2
  with beef *sukiyaki*
    165–6, *165*
  buckwheat 63
  hiyamugi with dipping
    sauce 179
  soba with dipping sauce
    175–6, *175*
  somen with dipping
    sauce 178–9
  soup *soba* noodles with
    chicken 176–7
  soup *udon* noodles with
    simmered bean curd
    177–8
  uses of 62
  wheat 62–3
nori seaweed 16, 61

oil
  omega-3 16
  temperature for frying
    27
  uses of 66
oil draining rack 24
oil skimmer 23
okra, blanched 82–3, *82*
omega-3 fats 16
omelette pan 23
omelettes *see* eggs
onions
  and potato soup 89–90
  see also spring onions
orange, green tea bavarois
  with 188

panko breadcrumbs 61
peas
  with boiled quails' eggs
    and spring onions
    87–8, *87*
  with braised beef and
    potatoes 155–6, *156*
  with chicken 142–3,
    143
  with steamed rice and
    chicken 172–3
  steamed rice with green
    (jade rice) 90, *90*
perilla 59
pickle
  Chinese cabbage 184–5
  Daikon radish in *yuzu*
    sweet vinegar 184
  plums (*umeboshi*) 67
  sweet and sour cabbage
    and cucumber 185
plums, pickled (*umeboshi*)
  67

ponzu sauce 43
porcelain 6
pork
    braised belly in miso
        157
    and choy-sum in miso
        sauce 159–60
    cutlets (on rice) 170
    deep-fried
        breadcrumbed loin
        (*tonkatsu*) 158–9, *159*
    loin with ginger-
        flavoured soy sauce
        160–1, *161*
    simmered loin with
        mustard soy sauce
        162–3, *162*
    and vegetable miso soup
        181–2, *181*
potato starch 66
potatoes
    braised beef with
        155–6, *156*
    and onion miso soup
        89–90
    sweet 57
poultry *see* chicken; duck
prawns
    futomaki rolls 94–6,
        95–6
    grilled tofu squares with
        dengaku miso sauce
        109–10
    savoury custard cup
        125–6, *125*
    scattered sushi (Osaka
        style) 69, 72–3
    skewered 30
    temaki rolls 98–9
    tempura 1, 128–9, *129*,
        173–4, 178
presentation of food 6, 8

quails' eggs, stir-fried with
    sugarsnap peas and
    spring onions 87–8,
    87

radish *see Daikon* radish;
    white radish
rectangle cutting technique
    29
regional cooking 9–10
rice
    central role of 6
    chicken and egg on
        steamed 167
    chicken, salmon and egg
        on 171–2, *171*
    cooling tub 22
    deep-fried
        breadcrumbed pork
        cutlets on (*katsu-don*)
        170

glutinous 48–9
glutinous with adzuki
    beans 168
grilled teriyaki chicken
    on (*kiji don*) 168–9,
    169
jade 90, *90*
shiitake mushroom
    84–5, *84*
steamed 79
steamed with chicken
    and vegetables 172–3
for sushi 91–2, *91*
tea-flavoured 173
tempura on 173–4
varieties of 48–9
rice bran 49
rice cakes, glutinous 49
rice cooker 23
rice paddle 22

sake 47
salmon
    with chicken and egg on
        rice 171–2, *171*
    futomaki rolls 94–6,
        95–6
    grilled marinated with
        Daikon radish 80–1,
        80
    temaki rolls 98–9
    teriyaki 139–40, *139*
salt 16, 17
sanbai-zu (three-flavoured
    vinegar) dressing 42
sansho powder 64
sardines simmered with
    ginger 136
sashimi
    beef 154–5, *154*
    filleting for 35–6
    knife 22
    mackerel 137–8, *138*
    recipes for 137–8
    slicing technique 36–7
sauces
    ground sesame 43–4
    miso 44
    ponzu 43
    soy 45
    see also stock; vinegar
        dressing
seafood *see* prawns; squid
seasonal factors 3, 7
seaweed
    health benefits of 16
    see also hijiki seaweed;
        konbu (kelp); *nori*
        seaweed; *wakame*
        seaweed
service of food 6, 8
sesame oil 66
sesame sauce 43–4
sesame seeds 64

sesame soy sauce 45
seven-spice pepper 64
shallow-frying 26
shamoji (rice paddle) 22
shari see sushi
shiitake mushrooms
    with chicken 142–3, *143*
    with chicken, salmon and
        egg on rice 171–2, *171*
    chicken stuffed 151–2
    with cod fillets 131–2,
        132
    health benefits of 16
    pork and vegetable miso
        soup 181–2, *181*
    rice and 84–5, *84*
    simmered (for sushi)
        92–3
    with steamed rice and
        chicken 172–3
    stir-fried with bean
        sprouts and spring
        onions 75
    tempura 128–9, *129*
    uses of 56, *56*
    vegetarian *dashi* stock
        40–1
    yakitori 149–50, *149*
shimeji mushrooms 56–7
shira-taki (thread
    konnyaku) 67
shiratama-ko powder 49
shiso leaves 19, 59
shojin-ryori cuisine 5–6, 8
simmering 25
slicing *sashimi* 36–7
soba noodles 63, 175–6,
    175, 176
sodium 16, 17
somen noodles 63, 178–9
soup
    beaten egg soup 73
    chicken broth 78–9, *78*
    Daikon radish and fried
        bean curd 180
    pork and vegetable miso
        181–2, *181*
    potato and onion miso
        89–90
    sesame-flavoured miso
        with vegetables and
        tofu 182–3
    tofu and *wakame* miso
        83–4, *83*
soy sauce 45, 46
soya beans
    in Buddhist cookery 5
    green 54
    health benefits of 11–12
    kinako 51
    natto 15, 51
    yuba 5, 51
    see also tofu
soya milk 5

spinach
    blanched 114–15, *114*
    and Chinese leaves roll
        116–17, *116*
    mustard– 54
    uses of 57
spring onions
    stir-fried with boiled
        quails' eggs and peas
        87–8, *87*
    stir-fried with shiitake
        mushrooms and bean
        sprouts 75
    uses of 57
square omelette pan 23
squash, *kabocha* 54,
    120–1, *121*
squid *tempura* 128–9, *129*,
    173–4
steamed rice 79
steaming 27–8
stem ginger 57
stir-fries
    bean sprouts, shiitake
        mushrooms and spring
        onions 75–6
    beef with ground *sansho*
        pepper 164
    boiled quails' eggs,
        sugarsnap peas and
        spring onions 87–8, *87*
    carrots with chilli 81–2,
        81
    method for 26
stock
    chicken 41
    primary *dashi* 38–9
    secondary *dashi* 39–40
    vegetarian *dashi* 40–1
structure, of meal 18
sudachi citron 65, *65*
sukiyaki 10, 165–6, *165*
sushi
    bo-zushi (stick sushi) 8
    chirashi-zushi (scattered
        sushi) 8, 9
    cucumber rolls 97–8
    development of 8–9
    futomaki rolls 94–6, 95–6
    golden thread eggs 93
    hako-zushi (box sushi) 8
    inari-zushi (vegetarian
        sushi) 8
    kanpyo 93
    Kyoto-style 9
    maki-zushi (rolled sushi)
        8, 9
    nigiri-zushi (hand-formed
        sushi) 8–9, 99–101,
        100–1
    omelette with
        mushrooms (*chakin-
        zushi* and *fukusa-zushi*)
        102–3, *102*

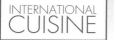

sushi *continued*
  Osaka-style 9
  oshi-zushi (pressed sushi)
    8
  rice for 22, 91–2, *91*
  rice in fried tofu
    pouches (*inari-zushi*)
    103–4, *103*
  scattered (Osaka style)
    69, 72–3
  simmered shiitake
    mushrooms 92–3
  temaki rolls 98–9
sushi mat 23
sweet potatoes 57
sweet vinegar dressing 42–3

takuwan 57–8
tamari soy sauce 46
tea
  ceremony 5, 6–8
  flavoured steamed rice
    173
  soba noodles 63
  see also green tea
techniques *see* cutting
    techniques; filleting;
    gutting
temaki rolls 98–9
tempura
  frying technique 27
  with noodles 175, 177,
    178
  on rice 173–4
teriyaki chicken *1, 18,*
    74–5, 168–9, *169*

teriyaki salmon 139–40, *139*
three-flavoured vinegar
    dressing 42
tofu
  and braised beef in
    sweet miso 105–6
  and braised *hijiki*
    seaweed 106
  chilled squares 107
  deep-fried 50
  deep-fried squares with
    dashi stock 108–9,
    108
  dried 50
  ganmodoki 5
  grilled bean curd 50
  grilled squares with
    dengaku miso sauce
    109–10
  health benefits of 11–12
  pouches with stuffed
    sushi rice 103–4, *103*
  simmered squares 110
  steak with Japanese
    mushrooms and ginger
    sauce *85*, 86
  and steamed white fish
    140–1, *140*
  thick fried bean curd 50
  uses of 49–50
  and vegetables in white
    miso sauce 110–11
  and *wakame* miso soup
    83–4, *83*
  yuba 5, 51

see also age (fried bean
    curd)
tonkatsu 143–4, 158, 170
tools
  cooking 22–4
  knives 21–2
trefoil 58
trout (scattered sushi
    Osaka style) *69*, 72–3
tsukune (minced chicken
    balls) 150
tuna (*nigiri-zushi* hand-
    formed sushi) 8–9,
    99–101, *100–1*
turnips 58
two-flavoured vinegar
    dressing 41–2

udon noodles 62, 165–6,
    165, 177–8
umeboshi (pickled red
    plums) 67

vegetable cutters 23
vegetable knife 21
vegetable peaks *30*
vegetable slicers 22–3
vegetables
  with chicken 142–3,
    143
  and pork miso soup
    181–2, *181*
  standard cuts for 28–9
  with steamed rice and
    chicken 172–3

in tofu and white miso
    sauce 110–11
vegetarian *dashi* stock
    40–1
vinegar, Japanese rice 47
vinegar dressing
  blanched okra with
    82–3, *82*
  chicken and cucumber in
    115
  with cucumber and
    wakame seaweed
    76–7, *76*
  sweet 42–3
  three-flavoured 42
  two-flavoured 41

wakame seaweed
  and cucumber with
    Japanese vinegar
    dressing 76–7, *76*
  health benefits of 16
  and simmered bamboo
    shoots 118–19
  and tofu soup 83–4, *83*
  uses of 62
wasabi 65, 112
wheat gluten 59–60
white radish 57
wood ear mushrooms 58

yakitori 149–50, *149*
yams, uses of 54
yuba 5, 51
yuzu citron 65, *65*, 184